Holistic
Wellbeing Method

Achieve ultimate health and wellness through nutrition and lifestyle changes

Includes 50 clean eating recipes

Sharon Pitman and Lorraine Pitman

ISBN: 978-1-326-44638-3

PublishNation, London
www.publishnation.co.uk

Acknowledgements

We would like to thank all who have supported us in writing this book. In particular, we would like to express our gratitude to our Mum and Stuart. Thanks to both of you for your belief that we could succeed. Thanks also to our readers. We sincerely hope that within these pages you will find something of significance to help you along your wellbeing journey.

Dedicated to our dad, James Pitman.

Contents

Introduction

Here at Holistichem, we believe that wellbeing is essential. Our body and mind is capable of great things. However, we often take them for granted yet still expect them to work perfectly. Boosting your wellbeing can help put you back on track towards optimum health.

Following the information provided in this book can help you reduce stress, increase energy, boost the immune system, maintain a healthy weight, lessen aches and pains, improve digestion and skin and much more. We know it works; we can see the difference it has made in our lives and want you to experience this as well.

How do you boost your wellbeing? Well, that is what we are here for. We have developed the Holistichem Wellbeing Method, a plan that we outline in this book. Through the information given, we will help you to incorporate simple, achievable lifestyle changes that will positively help you to change the way you look, feel, eat and think. We believe that complementary therapy is one of the best ways to ensure good wellbeing. This holistic plan encourages you to eat a healthy, wholefood diet and include rest, recreation, relaxation and positive thinking in your daily life. All of this helps to reduce stress. By reducing stress, we give our body and mind the best chance of functioning at its peak level.

In the pages that follow, we will give you lots of tips and advice about nutrition and wellbeing. It is amazing the positive changes that can take place when you make the commitment to look after yourself and take care of what you put into your body and mind. The old adage "a healthy body equals a healthy mind" is very true. When we do the best for our body and mind, we can make many improvements to our quality of life including how we look and feel. Without good health and wellbeing, we can't operate at our optimum. Every one of us is an individual. Depending on your current state of health, some of us have more needs than others.

1

However, that doesn't stop us from making improvements. As you begin to transform your lifestyle for the better, you will undoubtedly see positive changes and begin to feel healthier and more relaxed.

Our advice may not offer a complete cure for everyone, but it provides the tools to help make you feel better whatever your personal circumstances and also reduce the risk of things going wrong. You will soon see that making small lifestyle changes can improve our wellbeing in a big way. So, what are you waiting for? Let's get started by looking at the areas we will address:

   Eat a healthy, wholefood diet

   Achieve restful sleep and take regular exercise

   Make time to consciously relax

   Think and feel positive

A Word About Stress

Before we begin, let's have a closer look at stress and its effects on our body and mind. Stress has become commonplace. It has made its way into our everyday language. How many times do we describe a situation as being "stressful" or ourselves as "stressed"? Most of us, if not all, have experienced stress at some point due to either our personal life or work environment and even health conditions. Our increasingly busy lives make us susceptible to excessive stress.

Stress is simply the inability to cope with pressure. We all need a certain amount of pressure in our lives. Without it, we would not be able to undertake risks, meet challenges or be motivated. We need a certain amount of stress to live a fulfilling life. However, when we have too much pressure in our life the feelings of stress can spiral out of control. Long-term stress can lead to physical, mental and emotional problems such as poor immunity, raised blood pressure, low energy, muscle tension, headaches, poor concentration, irritability, anxiety and poor sleep. Left untreated, stress can lead to eventual burnout. As you can see, it is very important to keep stress at a healthy level.

You may have heard of the term "fight or flight"; this is an innate human response. When we are stressed, the body naturally produces this response. The body becomes alert and our muscles become tense and ready for action. The blood flow alters and redirects our hormones to allow us to either confront or flee the stressor. This was most effectively used by our cavemen ancestors who regularly faced dangerous and stressful situations in their role as hunter-gatherers. For example, when they made the decision to confront or run from a wild animal their bodies dealt with the situation using the fight or flight response, after said danger had passed their bodies then reverted to its natural relaxed state. Thankfully, nowadays we do not often face such perilous situations. Stress can help us react faster, provide strength and activate the body when needed. However, as most of our stress occurs from non-life threatening situations, we tend not to fully use the fight or flight response, leaving our bodies tense and mind under constant pressure.

Although you might not think so, your diet can also contribute to your stress levels. Dietary choices, such as refined and stimulating food and drink, puts the body's system under stress. Stress causes a rise in cortisol that makes us more prone to craving and overeating as well as causing inflammation. We need to follow a healthy diet so that we don't overburden our body's intricate function. Processed foods put pressure on the liver and kidneys to work harder to rid the body of unwanted toxins. These organs are essential for elimination, so we want them to work as effectively as possible. Put simply, poor diet makes it harder for them to do their job properly. For example, eating too much sugar causes changes in blood sugar levels, puts the pancreas under strain, causes mood swings and uses up stress-busting B vitamins. This is not to mention that it can also cause tooth decay, yeast overgrowth, increased risk of hypoglycaemia and diabetes as well as contributing to weight gain. Phew!

We can't always control the things that make us stressed, but we can control how we react. By changing your diet, thinking, lifestyle and how you relax, you can begin to take control of stress and regain vibrant wellbeing. Here goes...

Diet

The nutritional aspect of the Holistichem Wellbeing Method is based on a wholefood diet. This consists of eating clean, fresh and pure foods that will enable the body to function at its optimum. It also assists the healing process within the body. The aim of a wholefood diet is to eat a wide variety of fresh, unrefined foods whilst limiting processed and refined foods. Processed and refined foods, such as cakes, biscuits and junk food, have no nutritional value and can be detrimental to health. You will notice that we don't count calories, avoid fat or recommend "diet" foods. We believe in clean eating and know that eating "real" food, which never contains processed ingredients or artificial additives, benefits health and wellbeing. A wholefood diet also encourages natural weight loss. The body can store surplus fat, some of which is excess fluid. We tend to find that when we eliminate/reduce certain products, especially wheat and sugar, from our diet the unwanted fat naturally reduces. Once we reach our ideal weight, a wholefood diet will also help us maintain this. Of course, if you don't need to lose weight, don't worry; your weight will remain within healthy limits. Also, remember that we all react differently to food. What suits one person doesn't always suit another. Use the following suggestions as guidelines to build a healthy, wholefood diet. There is no "one size fits all" diet. Eat sensibly and do what feels right for you. We don't advocate restrictive eating and we will only advise you to remove certain foods if you have an intolerance/allergy. We like to take a balanced approach to diet and encourage you to adapt the information we give to suit you.

You will also notice that we recommend that, where possible, you eat organic food as it is grown without pesticides and toxins. Animal produce has often been produced using hormones that can add to the toxic load in our bodies. However, we do realise that organic is more expensive and, whilst it is not compulsory to eat this way, we would recommend it as a lifestyle choice if you can comfortably afford to do so. Also, depending on where you live, it isn't always easy to access an organic variety of absolutely every food type. We would rather you ate a wide variety of quality fresh food than avoid, for example, eating fruit and vegetables just because they are not organic. Aim to eat a varied wholefood diet and, where possible, opt for organic varieties. It may be useful to keep in mind that some fruits and vegetables are known to have more chemical and pesticide residue present in them. Apples, grapes, strawberries, peaches, nectarines, cucumber, celery, spinach, potatoes, peppers, tomatoes and chilli peppers are often known as the "dirty dozen". Where possible, it is best to eat organic varieties of these. There is also a group of fruit and vegetables known as the "clean fifteen" and these naturally contain less chemical and pesticide residue. These are kiwis, grapefruit, melon, mango, avocado, pineapple, papaya, sweet potatoes, asparagus, aubergine, peas, cabbage, onions, sweetcorn and mushrooms. Non-organic varieties can be eaten if it is not feasible to buy these organically grown. When eating non-organic produce, it is best to peel the outer skin, if possible, as this will help reduce some of the pesticides. Organic fruit and vegetables don't always need to be peeled, so if it is the type of produce that can be eaten with the skin on, such as carrots and apples, you can do so knowing that it has been grown without the use of pesticides.

The basis of a wholefood diet is as follows:

Eat lots of fresh fruit and vegetables. Depending on where you live, guidelines may vary for each country. An average of anywhere between five to seven portions per day is recommended. A minimum of two portions of fruit and three to five portions of vegetables is a good balance. You can, of course, eat more than this. The more plant foods you can consume, the better. For this reason, try to include as many fruit and vegetables as possible as they contain lots of vitamins, minerals and antioxidants. One adult portion weighs approximately 80g. For example, a portion is equivalent to one banana, two small kiwis, seven strawberries or three heaped tablespoons of peas. Remember, potatoes don't usually count as a vegetable portion. They are a good source of vitamin C and fibre but are very starchy. Always eat potatoes alongside other vegetables to boost your vegetable count. Opt for potatoes in their skins for the richest source of vitamins and fibre. This also helps break down carbohydrates more slowly. However, sweet potatoes do count as a vegetable portion. Eat lots of leafy green vegetables as these are especially rich in vitamins and minerals. Incorporate fruit and vegetables into every meal such as homemade smoothies, soup, dips, pasta sauce and salad.

Try steaming vegetables instead of boiling to retain vitamins. In general, try to avoid frying. Grilling, baking and poaching are healthier options. If you do fry, opt for unrefined, heat stable oils such as coconut oil, ghee or rapeseed. If you want to eat chips, try making your own healthy chips baked in the oven using the minimum of good quality oil.

Try to eat some raw fruit and vegetables every day. Enzymes, which are vital for health, are found only in fresh, raw fruit and vegetables. These enzymes are lost during cooking as heat destroys them. Including raw food in your diet provides the body with a quality supply of vitamins and minerals. Eating fruit and vegetables in their raw state provides the body with energy and helps to aid detoxification. Raw plant foods are cleansing and alkalising as well as beneficial for digestion. A fresh apple or a bowl of salad counts as raw food. Other easy raw food snacks are carrot sticks, cherry tomatoes, sliced peppers, avocados, etc. Smoothies and freshly squeezed juices are also a good source of raw food that you can easily incorporate into your diet. Raw food doesn't always have to be cold. You can gently warm up raw fruit and vegetables to approximately 48°C/118°F without destroying the enzymes. If you have a high-speed blender, you can easily whizz up some raw soups that are hot to the taste. You can use a dehydrator to warm raw foods too. This can add some variety and is especially good in colder climates. Of course, you don't need to have these gadgets. You can also get lots of raw goodness by simply enjoying fresh, uncooked fruit and vegetables.

Eat regular portions of unrefined grains. A portion is equivalent to approximately 50g uncooked grains or one slice of bread. Refined grains, such as white flour, white bread and processed breakfast cereals, are valueless. Switching to unrefined grains, such as wholemeal flour and wholewheat, provides complex carbohydrates, fibre, more vitamins and minerals and is beneficial to the heart and digestive tract. Healthy digestion is essential for good health. It is estimated that over half the immune system resides in the gut meaning that digestion plays a major role in immunity. Complex carbohydrates release sugar into the body at a much slower rate, helping to balance blood sugars and keeping us fuller for longer. Try introducing wholewheat pasta, rye crispbreads, rice cakes, brown rice and wholemeal bread, including seeded varieties. You may also like to try products made using spelt flour, barley flour, quinoa, bulgur wheat and oats. Try varying your unrefined grains. For example, you may try eating one portion of wholewheat daily, if tolerated, and then opt for other suggested alternative grains. If you have a gluten intolerance, opt for low or non-gluten varieties depending on the severity of your condition. Sprouted grains are rich in enzymes and nutrients. These varieties, such as sprouted oats, wholewheat and buckwheat, are also easily digested and are useful to add to your diet. This applies also to sprouted pulses, nuts and seeds. If you find it hard to digest grains, you may wish to avoid or keep them to a minimum, eating only varieties that are free from gluten/wheat.

Gluten and wheat intolerance is becoming increasingly common and can cause health problems such as allergies, respiratory issues and digestive upset. All gluten-free foods are free from wheat, but wheat-free foods are not always free from gluten. For example, wholemeal flour is free from refined wheat but still contains gluten. If an intolerance to gluten is present, it is best to avoid or limit your exposure. Some individuals have an allergy to wheat or gluten and/or coeliac disease, which means that a total avoidance of gluten is necessary. As well as the health aspect, many people find that reducing wheat and/or gluten can help them lose weight as it reduces bloating. The consumption of refined grains and processed foods can add to unwanted inches around the waist and other parts of the body. There is no need to avoid wheat completely unless you are sensitive to it, but we would advise that you don't overload on it and eat small, sensible quantities of unrefined varieties only.

Most supermarkets and health food shops now stock some gluten and wheat-free alternatives. Gluten-free breads, flours and pastas are widely available. Whilst gluten-free products are becoming more accessible, please be aware that gluten-free varieties are not always healthier. Many gluten-free products are processed. For example, biscuits and cakes still contain ingredients such as sugar. Indeed, some gluten-free produce have higher levels of sugar to compensate for the difference in texture that results from using gluten-free flours, etc. As always, try to eat as unprocessed as possible whether gluten/wheat is present or not.

A variety of grains are available that are suitable for those with a gluten/wheat sensitivity such as rice, buckwheat, amaranth, millet, tapioca, quinoa and corn. When using corn-based products, opt for non-GMO varieties. If you are sensitive to wheat only, you may still eat foods made from oats, rye, spelt and barley, etc. Some people who have a gluten intolerance can tolerate small amounts of foods that are lower in gluten such as those made with spelt, oats, etc. Similarly, you may be able to tolerate small amounts of wholemeal flour, bread, pasta, etc. However, we do not recommend this for those with coeliac disease. Gluten-free oats are available for those who can't tolerate standard varieties of oats. Each individual reacts differently and you will be able to assess how your body reacts to each grain. Obviously, if you have a diagnosed intolerance, we advise that you discuss this with your healthcare provider before trying any products containing gluten/wheat.

It is worth noting that some people find grains hard to digest. We believe that grains are good for you and are very healthy. However, they can be tough on the digestive system. Gluten-free or low-gluten grains tend to be tolerated better, especially if you have digestive problems and are essential if you have a gluten intolerance. Soaking grains, as well as beans, pulses, nuts and seeds, can be helpful as they contain an anti-nutrient known as phytic acid that can reduce the availability of some of the minerals which they naturally contain. This means that the body can't absorb these nutrients. Soaking these overnight removes the phytic acid, which allows the body to absorb nutrients, also making them easier to digest. If grains cause problems, it may be best to keep them to a minimum. You may find that your digestion improves by reducing or removing them from your diet. If you eat grains minimally, you may find that after a while you are gradually able to increase the amount you can comfortably eat. Wholegrains provide essential vitamins, minerals and fibre, so if you choose to restrict these please ensure that you obtain these nutrients from other sources such as fruit and vegetables.

It is possible to avoid grains completely on a long-term basis without any detrimental effect on health. Some people choose to follow a similar diet to that eaten by cavemen in Palaeolithic times, focusing on foods such as fruit, vegetables, nuts, seeds, eggs, fish and meats whilst avoiding grains, potatoes, legumes, dairy and sugar. Known as a Paleo diet, this is considered a primitive, unprocessed style of eating. Our diets have certainly changed due to industrial methods that have allowed us to produce grains, such as wheat, which was unheard of in primal times. As a result, heavily processed foods have become the norm. Some people genuinely fare better if they remove grains, including healthy, unrefined grains. This tends to benefit people with digestive problems and/or overactive immune systems. Should you choose to avoid all grains, you may like to try grain-free almond and coconut flour as a replacement for conventional flour. Whilst it is feasible to eat this way indefinitely, it is also very restrictive. We don't want your healthy eating regime to be challenging, so always follow the wholefood diet outlined. If you wish to fine-tune your diet to suit your body's needs, then please do so. You may wish to reduce your grain consumption if you feel this helps when any unwanted digestive and associated inflammatory symptoms flare-up.

If you have problems with certain foods, it may be that you have a food intolerance. You can be intolerant to virtually any food, but the most common intolerances are foods such as wheat, gluten, dairy, soy, yeast and corn. Another food sensitivity is FODMAPs. This stands for Fermentable Oligosaccharides Disaccharides Monosaccharides and Polyols. These short chain carbohydrates are poorly digested or absorbed by the small intestine and are found in gluten, lactose, fructose, etc. For example, FODMAPs occur naturally in foods such as apples, mango, pears, onions, avocado, asparagus, pulses, garlic, honey, xylitol and agave nectar. These can often cause irritable bowel syndrome and digestive symptoms. Not every food high in FODMAPs will cause everyone problems. You may be able to eat some with no digestive problems and others you may be able to eat in moderation. A lot of foods that are high in FODMAPs are very healthy and should only be restricted if they cause problems for you. For example, onions, leeks and garlic are rich in antioxidants. However, they can also prove troublesome for those sensitive to FODMAPs. You can easily substitute these if you require to use them in cooking. You can replace onions with the green part of spring onions or use chives instead. These are often better tolerated. Whilst the white part of a leek is usually used, you can use the green part instead as this is lower in FODMAPs. Likewise, garlic can be replaced with a garlic-infused oil. This provides the flavour without any unpleasant side effects. Honey, xylitol and agave nectar are all natural sweeteners, but these too can be problematic. If this is the case, these can be replaced with coconut sugar, maple syrup and brown rice syrup, also known as rice malt syrup, instead. As with most food sensitivities, you can find alternatives that are suitable for your personal needs. Remember, you can use these substitutes in any of the recipes later in this book.

Symptoms of food intolerance include digestive issues, congestion, headaches, etc. In order to identify food intolerances, you must methodically remove each food group from your diet. We would not recommend that you remove too many food groups at any one time. It is best to restrict one food type at a time. This allows you to accurately observe the effect of removing and reintroducing each food type whilst not limiting your diet and nutritional intake. For two weeks, you should avoid eating a specific food group. For example, you may wish to start by avoiding all products containing gluten. You may notice that you feel better within a few days. However, you really do need to continue avoidance for two weeks to fully identify whether this food group is problematic. After two weeks of avoidance, you should now reintroduce the food to your diet. Don't eat this food every day. Include it in your diet a few times per week, for example, approximately every four days. Diet is a very personal thing and what suits you may not necessarily suit others. It is always advisable to try and identify what works best for you. If a certain food or drink upsets your digestion or causes other symptoms, avoid or limit this.

Eat good quality free-range eggs only. Where possible, buy organic as non-organic may contain synthetic hormones. Eggs are a good source of protein and vitamin B12 and are an essential part of the diet, especially if no meat is eaten. Many people think that eggs are bad for the cholesterol level. This is, in fact, a myth and they can be eaten without any detrimental effect on cholesterol levels. Eggs are ideal at breakfast and as a healthy snack. You can also make a healthy egg replacement using flax or chia seeds. These are a great option for vegans or those who have an allergy to eggs. It is also useful for baking if you wish to add healthy seeds to your recipe or if you have run out of eggs. Simply mix one tablespoon ground flax or chia seeds with three tablespoons water. Stir well and let sit for 15 minutes, preferably in the fridge. This mixture can be used to replace one egg; if you need two eggs for a recipe, you can double the quantities.

Eat oily fish. Approximately two portions of fish per week is recommended, one of which should be oily fish. This provides omega-3 fatty acids. Oily fish helps to reduce inflammation in the system and is beneficial for the heart, hormones, immune system and problem skin. Salmon, fresh tuna, trout and mackerel are all examples of oily fish and should be included in the diet on a regular basis. Whilst we don't want lots of fat in our diet, we should be aiming to include healthy monounsaturated and polyunsaturated fats. These are good fats that help to keep us healthy and can contribute to a lower cholesterol level and a strong heart and immune system. If you are vegetarian/vegan, you can also obtain omega-3 fatty acids from flax, hemp and chia seeds. These beneficial fatty acids are also present in walnuts, soybeans and leafy green vegetables such as spinach. When eating fish, where possible, try to buy organic/wild and sustainable varieties.

Include pulses such as lentils and beans. Approximately three heaped tablespoons count as one vegetable portion. These are a good source of protein and fibre. Eating houmous regularly is a great way to get pulses into your diet. It is an excellent healthy food that is ideal as a snack with rice cakes or as a lunchtime meal spread on a baked potato. Try combining some pulses with wholegrains, such as brown rice, to provide complete vegetable protein. Meat contains all the amino acids needed for building health. However, vegetarian sources are incomplete proteins, as they don't contain every amino acid. There are some exceptions to this, such as quinoa, which is a complete protein. Eating pulses and grains together ensures that the body gets all the amino acids it needs. This is useful to remember when eating vegetarian meals. It is possible to obtain adequate amino acids if you eat a wide variety of pulses and grains. Don't worry too much if you do not always combine pulses with grains. The body is capable of making its own complete protein if a variety of foods is eaten throughout the day. You may also like to add Bragg Liquid Aminos to your diet. This is a condiment that is rich in amino acids and tastes similar to soy sauce and tamari. It is derived from non-GMO soybeans and contains naturally occurring sodium. You may wish to add a small amount to your diet, but avoid this if you have been advised to follow a no salt/sodium diet by your healthcare provider. If you are unable to tolerate pulses, you may have to keep consumption to a minimum or try soaking them before cooking as this can make digestion easier. If pulses cause a lot of digestive distress, it may be best to avoid them. If you wish, you can always try reintroducing them later to see if you tolerate them better.

Include vegetarian-based products in your diet. A wholefood diet mainly consists of fresh vegetables and fruit as well as pulses and wholegrains. The emphasis should be on eating less meat and more fruit and vegetables. People who eat meat in moderation and those who are vegetarian/vegan tend to be healthier and reduce their risk of ill health and disease. There is nothing wrong with eating good quality animal produce, if ethically acceptable to the individual. However, the healthiest diets keep meat intake to a minimum. If you do eat animal produce, taking a flexitarian approach is a good idea as the main source of your diet is plant-based with occasional meat and fish intake. Remember, there are products available, including Quorn and tofu, which can be used as meat alternatives. They tend to be naturally low in fat and a good source of protein. Please be aware that not all pre-prepared vegetarian/vegan foods are healthy. Just like any other processed food, they can often contain sugar, wheat and/or gluten. Always pay attention to the ingredient listing on products or, better still, prepare meals yourself in order to avoid processed ingredients. Watch out for foods containing soy as this can cause intolerance or allergy in some individuals. Soy is rich in phytoestrogens, however, can cause problems in some women with hormonal conditions and may cause unwanted flare-ups of symptoms. Additionally, excessive soy consumption can suppress thyroid function that may adversely affect an underactive thyroid. In such cases, soy should be used with caution and it really is a case of seeing how it works for each person. If you can tolerate soy, as with everything, consume in moderation. You can enjoy a tofu-based meal regularly. However, you should include a range of vegetarian sources of protein to add variety to your diet. Opt for non-GMO, preferably organic, products such as tofu and soya milk. When eating soy, we recommend opting for fermented varieties of tofu, miso, tamari, etc. Limit soy intake to no more than twice per week to ensure the health benefits without any negative effects.

If you do limit or avoid meat, in particular the intake of red meat, you may have to watch out for low levels of iron. We advise that you only take iron supplements if you have a medically confirmed iron deficiency as it is important not to over supplement. You can obtain iron from plant sources such as leafy green vegetables and pulses. Eating iron-rich plant foods with vitamin C sources, such as kiwis or fresh orange juice, helps the body absorb non-animal source iron. If you also choose to avoid eggs in addition to dairy and meat, for example, due to veganism or allergy, you can obtain dietary source vitamin B12 from fortified wholegrain cereals, vegetarian foods and dairy-free milks. You may also like to add a vitamin B12 supplement to your diet.

For those who choose to eat meat, consider limiting red meat consumption. Eat no more than approximately two portions a week, less if possible. Red meat is a good source of iron but tends to be rich in saturated fats and can contribute to inflammation. If you do eat red meat, choose lean cuts of meat, such as beef or venison, as these are healthier. You don't need to avoid it completely, if you like red meat you can still enjoy it, just don't eat it excessively. Pork tends to be harder to digest and is often highly refined and very salty. Refined pork products, such as processed ham, should be avoided or limited. Many types of bacon and sausages are also made with processed ingredients. If you do wish to eat bacon, choose a variety that has at least 97% pork, no added water or sugar, preferably sustainably reared and free from nitrates. Likewise, choose sausages with a similar pork content and, if required, select gluten-free varieties. Opt for white meat, such as chicken and turkey, as these are leaner. Aim to eat no more than two portions or less of poultry per week as part of your wholefood diet. The less meat we eat, the cleaner our diet will be. Where possible, eat organic, grass-fed, pastured or naturally reared free-range varieties of meat as these are healthier and ethical options. Organic meat is free from hormones and added toxins. Grass-fed meat tends to be leaner and richer in healthy fats as opposed to animal produce that has been grain-fed. A portion of meat should be approximately the size and thickness of the palm of your hand.

Include unsaturated fats, such as extra virgin olive oil, as this is a good source of monounsaturated fatty acids and helps to lower cholesterol. These are anti-inflammatory, helping to maintain heart health and hormone balance. Use it in cooking or drizzle over salads as a dressing. Adding healthy oils to salads can actually help us to absorb a lot of the nutrients present in the vegetables. Unrefined, cold pressed and/or raw varieties are best. Coconut oil is another healthy fat and can be used in cooking and baking as well as spread on rice cakes and oatcakes. An avocado also contains healthy fats and is a great source of vitamin E. You can include traditional animal fats, such as ghee and duck/goose fat, if these are ethically acceptable. Although fat has often been given a bad reputation, these actually offer a healthy balance of fats and are safe to cook with at high temperatures.

Eat nuts and seeds. Nuts, such as unsalted, preferably raw, cashew nuts and Brazil nuts are all good sources of unsaturated fat, as are sunflower and pumpkin seeds. They have essential fatty acids and are a great source of protein. They are ideal sprinkled on salads, added to cereals and yoghurts or eaten as a snack. Try toasting seeds in a dry frying pan for a few minutes until golden brown to really bring out the flavour. Many nuts and seeds, such as walnuts, flax and sesame seeds, contain phytoestrogens. These have numerous benefits including antioxidant properties. They also help to balance hormonal health. Phytoestrogens also occur in a variety of fruits, vegetables, legumes and wholegrains such as berries, carrots, lentils and wheatgerm. By regularly eating nuts and seeds, you can increase your intake of healthy fats, antioxidants and phytoestrogens. If you have digestive problems, you may find nuts and seeds hard to digest. If so, try grinding them and adding them to smoothies or eat smooth varieties of unrefined nut butters. Of course, you can do this too, even if your digestion is fine. The digestive system does not break down whole flaxseed, also known as linseed. For this reason, always opt for ground flaxseed. Nuts and seeds are very healthy. Varieties such as chia seeds are soothing on the digestive tract as well as an excellent source of plant-based omega oils.

Reduce excessive dairy consumption, particularly cows' milk produce. You can eat dairy produce, such as natural yoghurt, preferably opting for organic and/or grass-fed varieties. Always make sure you eat unsweetened natural or Greek yoghurt as fruit flavoured ones tends to have sugar added. Cultured dairy, such as yoghurt and kefir, is generally well tolerated and may be consumed without any adverse effects due to the beneficial probiotic content. Unless you are allergic to dairy or are vegan, we always advise that you include cultured dairy in your diet due to their immense health benefits. They tend to be lower in lactose and most people can tolerate them in their diet. If you can't tolerate dairy, you can opt for non-dairy sources of probiotics. There are also a variety of yoghurts available made from non-dairy milk such as coconut yoghurt.

You can eat some butter as part of a wholefood diet. People have a tendency to think butter is bad for them and it does contain some saturated fat, but within limit, it is perfectly acceptable. Indeed, many commercial margarines and low-fat spreads contain additives and chemical ingredients. Subsequently, they are not as healthy as they are perceived to be. Butter is a natural source product and small quantities of good quality, preferably organic and/or grass-fed, butter is allowable. Likewise, good quality ghee is acceptable as it has anti-inflammatory properties. Both of these are also lower in lactose and usually well tolerated. If you don't eat any dairy produce, please ensure that any butter alternative you consume is good quality, free from additives and preferably organic. Raw coconut oil can also be used as a spread to replace butter. It contains healthy fat as well as natural anti-fungal properties that aid digestion.

Likewise, if you wish to include milk in the diet, you may opt for small amounts of organic and/or grass-fed whole milk. There is not a lot of difference between whole milk and semi-skimmed in their saturated fat level, therefore, small amounts of full-fat milk is acceptable. Lactose-free milk and A2 milk is easier to digest if milk usually causes you problems. Regular cows' milk contains both A1 and A2 protein. A1 protein can cause unwanted side effects such as digestive upset and congestion. However, A2 milk contains only A2 protein and is usually well tolerated. Raw milk is often better tolerated than pasteurised milk. It is also beneficial for immunity. However, as it is unpasteurised, only drink raw milk if you feel comfortable in doing so and always buy from a reliable supplier. Like all dairy produce, you can enjoy raw milk in moderation. If you are pregnant, it is advisable to avoid raw milk and products, such as cheese, that have been made using it. You may wish to include some cows' milk alternatives in your diet. Some people choose to avoid cows' milk completely, perhaps due to intolerance. Certainly, cows' milk can cause a lot of inflammation in the diet. It is also linked to allergies, respiratory issues and digestive problems. Good alternatives are goats', ewes', soya, oat, almond, coconut or rice milk produce. When selecting non-dairy milk, opt for unsweetened/naturally sweetened varieties and those free from carrageenan. This is a natural source ingredient that is sometimes present in dairy-free milk such as almond and coconut milk. Carrageenan is not digestible and can cause inflammation, particularly in the digestive system, so it is best to avoid any produce containing this.

Similarly, goats' and ewes' cheese, which are lower in lactose, can be consumed as part of a wholefood diet. For example, look out for halloumi and feta cheese made with goats' and ewes' milk instead of cows' milk. Remember, cheese contains a lot of fat, so should be eaten in moderation. A portion of cheese is approximately the size of a small matchbox. Hard, strong flavoured cheeses, such as Pecorino Romano that is made with ewes' milk, is a good alternative to Parmesan and can be grated to make a small amount go further. Cottage cheese is lower in saturated fat and is often well tolerated by those with digestive issues. Lactose-free milk products, such as cheese and yoghurt, are also suitable and are ideal for intolerances. Aim to include some healthy, calcium-rich dairy products or a suitable alternative each day. Try varying the type of dairy produce you eat for variety. This can also help to reduce possible intolerance to cows' milk. If you do choose to avoid dairy products, you can obtain calcium from foods such as leafy green vegetables, sesame seeds and chia seeds. If you do not eat any dairy products, perhaps due to intolerance, allergy or veganism, then you will obviously have to avoid all milk products, including ewes' and goats' produce. In this case, you can supplement your diet with a variety of dairy-free produce.

Include fermented foods in your diet. These are helpful for the digestive system and immunity. They are rich in natural source probiotics. Consuming fermented foods can increase the good bacteria in your gut. It has a healing effect on digestion and can help you digest food better. Fermented food has a lot of beneficial enzymes. The fermentation process helps effectively pre-digest the food so that the resulting cultured produce is easily digested. These enzymes also help you digest other foods that you eat at the same time as part of a meal. Fermented foods can help with all digestive conditions and even has a healing effect on conditions such as candida and leaky gut syndrome. They also contain a variety of vitamins and other nutrients. Remember, good digestion is important for a healthy immune system, so the inclusion of fermented foods can help to build immunity. In addition to cultured dairy produce, such as milk kefir and yoghurt, you can also consume a range of fermented drinks such as non-dairy water kefir and kombucha. Fermented vegetables, such as sauerkraut and kimchi, are beneficial too. You can buy ready-made cultured products or easily make your own. For example, kefir can be made at home using milk kefir grains in milk or water kefir grains in a solution of water and sugar. Likewise, kombucha is made using tea and sugar resulting in a sparkling drink that is rich in probiotics and good bacteria as well as gut healing glutamic acid. In order to make kombucha, you need to have a SCOBY (symbiotic colony of bacteria and yeast). This acts as the culture to ferment the sugary tea solution into a beneficial drink. The fermentation process effectively eats the sugar; therefore, you do not have to worry about excess sugar consumption. Any sugar that remains will be negligible. Kombucha that has been fermented for longer will have an even lower sugar content. Whilst beneficial, if you have a condition that affects your blood sugar levels, it is always advisable to speak to your healthcare provider when introducing kombucha. You can obtain kefir grains and kombucha cultures from reputable suppliers. These will usually come with full instructions as to how to make these probiotic drinks. These cultures are reusable and will multiply with every batch. This allows you to always have a supply and you can also share your grains and/or SCOBY with family and friends.

Limit sugar intake. If possible, avoid all refined sugar. Excessive sugar consumption causes blood glucose levels to spike, putting stress on the adrenal glands. It can also lead to excessive yeast growth within the body that can cause a multitude of digestive problems. Eating too much sugar contributes greatly to weight gain and can cause skin problems as well as increasing the risk of developing diabetes. Inflammatory conditions can be worsened by sugar. Simply reducing sugar can decrease associated symptoms. Limiting our sugar consumption is also better for our teeth as it can help prevent decay. Sugar is toxic stuff that can wreak havoc in the body. Refined sugar is found in chocolate, sweets, jam, cakes, biscuits, cereal bars, breakfast cereals, ready-meals, etc. Look out for hidden sugar as it can pop up in the most unexpected places. Watch out for ingredients such as maltodextrin, dextrose and high-fructose corn syrup as these are other names for sugar. Many varieties of refined sugar have also been genetically modified. Try cutting down on sugar by eating naturally sugar-free or low-sugar alternatives. Always choose unrefined varieties. Be wary of commercial "low-fat" or "sugar-free" food as they tend to be highly processed, often containing artificial sweeteners and additives. In fact, many processed low-fat foods often contain refined sugar. Look out for foods sweetened with natural sugars/substitutes such as fruit, honey, agave nectar, stevia, coconut sugar and xylitol. Where possible, opt for organic and/or raw varieties of sweeteners such as honey and agave nectar. When using xylitol, opt for sustainably sourced and non-GMO varieties. Although natural source sugars are much healthier, you still don't want to eat them all the time. Enjoy them occasionally as a clean treat, but it is best to ensure that they don't make up a huge part of your diet. Another form of sugar is raw cane sugar. This is unrefined and whilst it retains more minerals than processed sugar, it is still sugar, so you may wish to minimise your intake or avoid it completely. Opt for fresh fruit or foods made with natural sweeteners. Small amounts of raw, unrefined sugar is acceptable. If you do choose to eat unrefined sugar, where possible, opt for an organic variety and consume small amounts only.

It is also worth remembering that fruit contains natural sugar. Avocados and lemons are very low-sugar fruits, as are all berries, apples, kiwis and limes. There is no problem eating a banana, which is fairly high in sugar, but please realise they can cause spikes in your blood sugar. Similarly, grapes are also quite high in sugar. For this reason, it is best not to eat high-sugar fruits in excess. Although by all means, include plenty of fruit in your diet to boost your immunity. For example, bananas are a great source of fibre, potassium and vitamin B6, whilst grapes are rich in phytonutrients such as resveratrol. Dried fruit is very high in natural sugar, so you might want to keep an eye on how much of it you eat. As always, you don't need to avoid it, but you may want to keep consumption at a sensible level. Feel free to enjoy fibre-rich dried fruit, such as Medjool dates, as fruit is always going to be better for you than sugary sweets and snacks. The fibre in fruit helps the body to slow down the effect on blood sugar. Therefore, unless you have a health condition affecting your blood sugar, you don't need to exclude or limit your intake of fruits that are naturally higher in sugar. However, just make sure that you don't overdo it. Some people tolerate fruit better than others do. Excessive fruit consumption can cause digestive upset in some individuals. If this is the case, stick to one or two pieces per day, ensuring that you also eat plenty of vegetables. Always listen to your body to see how it reacts to food; then base your choices on this. Above all, keep sugar to an absolute minimum and preferably eat unrefined varieties only. Many people think it is impossible to go without their sweet treats, but opting for unrefined products made with healthy, natural sugars means that you do not need to deprive yourself of a little sweetness. As you reduce your sugar intake, you will notice that your sugar cravings will subside. You will soon be able to pass on sugar-laden cakes and enjoy healthier substitutes.

A lot of people worry about how they will deal with sweet cravings when reducing their sugar intake. Please be assured that this lessens the longer you avoid sugar. As you begin to introduce natural sweeteners, you will find that a small amount is all that is needed to satisfy. Should you ever choose to eat something containing regular sugar, once you have successfully reduced it in your diet, you will most likely find that it tastes extremely sweet and not particularly enjoyable. Whilst cutting down on sugar, you might find it helpful to include sweet flavoured vegetables in your main meal such as carrots, parsnips, sweet potatoes, butternut squash, pumpkin, sweetcorn, yellow peppers and sugar snap peas. These all have a natural sweetness that may help satisfy any cravings. Remember to include lots of leafy green vegetables also. You can also try adding spices to your cooking to provide satisfying flavour. Spices, such as cinnamon, can add a slightly sweet flavour to food and contains antioxidant and anti-fungal properties that, for example, can help strengthen the immune system and fight yeast overgrowth. Sprinkling some cinnamon over porridge or adding it to sugar-free home baking can provide a good alternative to sweeteners. Ginger is another versatile spice that also helps detoxify and has anti-inflammatory properties that can soothe inflammation in the digestive tract whilst easing aches and pains. Remember that fruit, in particular low-sugar/low to medium glycaemic fruit, such as cherries and kiwis, may be adequate to provide any desired sweetness. A bowl of plain, unsweetened, probiotic-rich, natural yoghurt served with some berries is an ideal alternative to dessert. You may find it helpful to drink palate cleansing teas, such as peppermint or other herbal teas, as this can satisfy and curb any sweet cravings. Small amounts of carob, which has a similar taste to chocolate, is a good alternative as long as you opt for unsweetened varieties. You don't even have to cut out chocolate, providing you choose quality, unprocessed varieties made with raw cacao. Raw chocolate contains nutrients and antioxidants. It tends to be made with natural, unrefined sweeteners, such as agave nectar and coconut sugar, and you can enjoy small amounts of raw chocolate.

Reduce salt intake. Eating too much salt increases the risk of cardiovascular disease and can cause fluid retention. Try using herbs and spices to season food. When using salt, opt for a good quality sea salt or pink Himalayan salt as these contain more minerals. Pink Himalayan salt has many health benefits. For example, it can help to balance PH levels and adrenal function. Watch out for added salt in foods. If using tinned vegetables, always choose those containing water with no added salt and sugar. You can also season food with small quantities of soy-based condiments such as tamari and Bragg Liquid Aminos. For a soy-free alternative, you can use coconut aminos. However, whilst you don't need to avoid it completely, remember to keep salt intake to a minimum.

Consider reducing excessive intake of foods containing yeast if you have yeast-related issues. Foods such as stock cubes, yeast extract spreads, some breads, mushrooms, Quorn and alcohol, contain yeast. Whilst they do not need to be removed completely and some are actually healthy, you may want to eat them in moderation or limit your intake to prevent yeast build-up. Too much yeast within the system can cause problems such as thrush or digestive imbalances. Yeast should only be avoided if you have a yeast intolerance/allergy or a long-term condition such as candidiasis. This can lead to persistent thrush, fatigue or immune dysfunction. Certainly, yeast is in a lot of our food and reducing our intake of it can allow the stomach to produce more good bacteria, therefore, protecting our digestive and immune system. Limit soy sauce and vinegar as these both can promote the growth of yeast. Instead, opt for gluten-free tamari and raw apple cider vinegar. Nutritional yeast is a savoury condiment that, contrary to its name, does not encourage the overgrowth of yeast within the body. It is a rich source of B vitamins, making it ideal for boosting this essential vitamin. It is also useful for those who avoid meat, dairy and eggs. Likewise, kefir and kombucha contain beneficial yeasts that are good for you. They are a useful addition to the diet and do not need to be avoided. You can also make your own healthy yeast and additive-free stock from vegetables. Simply boil vegetables in water with a bay leaf, whole black peppercorns and optional seasoning. Then simmer for at least 45 minutes. If you are a meat-eater, you can include bones from quality, organic and/or grass-fed/pastured meat. This adds nutrients, collagen and a source of good quality gelatine that provides healing properties for digestion, immunity, joint health and skin. Cook as above, however, bone broth will require to simmer for at least 4-6 hours. You can simmer for longer to extract as much goodness from the bones as possible. For example, chicken bones can be simmered for up to 24 hours and beef bones for up to 48 hours. You can use high quality fish bones too. Choose non-oily varieties and simmer for 2 hours only. You can also add two tablespoons of raw apple cider vinegar to bones, approximately 30 minutes before cooking, to help draw out beneficial minerals such as calcium and magnesium. As well as a stock, this broth provides a savoury drink and can be used to cook grains, pulses and vegetables in.

Drink fresh fruit and vegetable juice. Freshly squeezed is best. Shop-bought juice often contains sugar, so juice your own or ensure that you purchase good quality juice with no added sugar. Freshly squeezed juice is very therapeutic and packed with vitamins and minerals. Juices made from fresh fruit and vegetables, particularly green varieties of vegetables, increases the intake of live enzymes. They are also gentle on digestion. As these are liquefied, they are effectively pre-digested allowing the stomach to instantly absorb the nutrients present. This also removes the fibre from fruit and vegetables. Whilst it is important to include fibre in the diet, too much roughage can easily upset sensitive digestion. Remember, unless you have digestive problems, we always recommend that you include fibre in your diet for the many health benefits it provides. Approximately 150ml counts as one portion, but remember that drinking further glasses of the same juice does not count towards more portions. One glass of freshly squeezed juice counts towards your raw food intake. Remember, fruit juice also contains natural concentrated sugars. For this reason, it should be kept to a minimum. Most benefit is derived from eating the whole fruit as it is less concentrated and you get more fibre from it. Although freshly squeezed juice is still beneficial to the diet, it should be consumed alongside a variety of wholefoods. Try making fresh fruit juice with medium to low-sugar fruits and combining them with vegetables to help to control blood sugar levels. A good example of this is apple and carrot juice which most people find quite pleasant. A maximum of one glass of freshly squeezed fruit juice is ideal. You can dilute this with water, if desired. Try incorporating a variety of vegetable-based juices too. You can also try a smoothie made with fresh or frozen fruit, which gives you the added benefits of the fibre contained within the whole fruit. You may like to try green smoothies made with leafy green vegetables, fruit and water, which are rich in chlorophyll and fibre, helping slow down the absorption of sugar from fruit. When making green smoothies, the blending process effectively helps to break down the cellulose wall of the leafy vegetables. This means the fibre present is easier to digest. Fibre also helps to keep us regular and binds toxins, helping to flush them through our system. You can get plenty of fibre in your diet by eating a wide variety of fruit and vegetables. It is also present in foods such as wholegrains, oats, nuts and seeds.

Avoid or limit caffeine as this is a stimulant. It can cause palpitations, stress the adrenals and make you feel jittery. Caffeine is found in coffee, tea, soft drinks, chocolate and cocoa. Drink more water or try a coffee substitute such as those made with barley, rye, dandelion or chicory. Alternatively, you can drink herbal teas such as rooibos, peppermint and fruit teas. Green tea/white tea has a small amount of caffeine but has antioxidant properties. Decaffeinated varieties of green tea are also available. Approximately one to four cups a day is acceptable. Likewise, raw chocolate and raw cacao powder have small quantities of caffeine present. However, it also has lots of beneficial properties such as antioxidants, vitamins and minerals. Although raw cacao doesn't usually cause any problems, carob is free from caffeine and tastes similar, making it an ideal substitute. If you must drink coffee, try limiting yourself to one or two cups each day. Opt for decaffeinated varieties, choosing organic, where possible, to reduce any chemicals present. Adding a tablespoon of raw coconut oil, organic and/or grass-fed butter or ghee to coffee can increase the nutrient content and whilst it might sound unusual, it actually tastes pleasant. Limiting coffee is the best idea. If you can't bear the thought of eliminating it totally, try drinking it only as an occasional treat. Similarly, decaffeinated tea is always preferable. Like coffee, black tea can be enjoyed occasionally. If possible, opt for organic varieties. Coffee and tea do have some health benefits. They contain antioxidants, however, should still only be consumed minimally. Kombucha tea also contains small amounts of caffeine. This probiotic drink is very healthy and, like green tea, is beneficial. If caffeine is a concern for you, look for kombucha made with tea that is lower in caffeine such as green or white tea. Drink at least eight glasses of clean water per day. Filtered water is very pure and mineral water is also acceptable. Avoid tap water as it contains toxins. Try starting the day with hot water and a slice of lemon to refresh and aid detoxification. If you find it hard to drink water, you might like to try flavouring it naturally. Adding slices of cucumber and allowing it to infuse in chilled water is very refreshing. Similarly, you can do this with lemon, lime and mint leaves as well as a variety of fruits such as berries and oranges.

Limit alcohol intake. Alcohol contains lots of sugar and empty calories with no nutritional value. Processing it puts a strain on the liver. Keep alcohol to a minimum and, if possible, avoid completely. If you do choose to drink alcohol, do so only on occasion and, where possible, opt for organic and/or gluten-free varieties. Cigarettes are stimulants, extremely bad for health and also raise blood sugar levels. They should be avoided altogether.

By introducing more wholefoods into your diet, you should see a marked improvement in your energy levels, skin and digestion. It is important to eat regular meals, approximately five or six per day, of which three of them should be main meals and two or three should be snacks. Do what is best for you. For example, you can have an extra snack if you feel you need this. It is useful to get into the habit of eating protein, carbohydrate and alkaline foods as part of each meal. Remember, you can include some healthy fats too. Alkaline foods, such as fruit and vegetables, help reduce the acid in our diet. We all have acid in our system and when there is too much it can cause inflammation, problems with the digestive system and, in general, ill health. By all means, do not exclude acid foods such as meat, fish, nuts and seeds. All of these can be very beneficial to health, but including more alkaline foods, such as leafy green vegetables, salads, avocados, lemons and almonds, helps create a favourable balance within the system. A good rule is to remember that vegetables should take up at least half of an average sized dinner plate.

By eating proteins and carbohydrates together, you can help to control blood sugar levels. Protein slows down sugar uptake. Carbohydrates are essentially sugar. All carbohydrates will be converted to sugar. Even complex carbohydrates, such as brown rice, will still be converted from starch to sugar in the system, albeit at a very slow rate. Therefore, complex carbohydrates are far more desirable than refined wheat, which just creates an instant sugar hit in the body. This is the reason why at times, if you are feeling hungry, you tend to reach for a biscuit to fill you up in between meals. This creates a sugar rush followed by a slump, which means we tend to eat more and can lead to weight gain. That is why it is important to always eat breakfast. Breakfast, as the word suggests, means to "break fast". We need to balance our sugar levels after not eating throughout the night, so by skipping breakfast or eating a refined meal, such as a bowl of sugary cereal, we just cause our sugar levels to rise and fall. This makes us more likely to snack on unhealthy foods throughout the morning to keep us going until lunchtime.

Where possible, opt for a healthy combination of foods. A good example of this would be to eat a rice cake with a spread of houmous. This is a healthy balance of carbohydrate and protein. Eat with a piece of fruit or slices of cucumber as a light meal or snack. This ideal snack will help to control your blood sugar, count towards your fruit and vegetable portion for the day and keep you going until the next meal. Nut butter and cottage cheese are other proteins that are great served on rice cakes. Rice cakes are low in fat, but as they are a carbohydrate, they can cause an instant increase in blood sugar that can just as easily lead to a dip in glucose levels. Combining them with a protein-rich food is ideal as they help to sustain blood sugar levels, helping to keep you feeling fuller for longer and preventing sugar crashes. Opting for seeded varieties of rice cakes can further help to slow down the release of carbohydrates. Fruits naturally contain some carbohydrates. Eating fruit with some protein helps to balance sugar levels. A portion of fruit, such as a fresh apple, eaten with protein-rich yoghurt is another healthy nutritious snack. Of course, you needn't worry if you eat a piece of fruit on its own. Obviously, this is very healthy. Naturally occurring fruit sugar is released more slowly than refined sugar. Whole fruit and its outer skin are rich in fibre, which can help slow down the release of natural sugar. Some people actually benefit from eating fruit alone, finding it easier to digest when eaten separately from other foods. Good sources of healthy carbohydrates are oatcakes, rice cakes, brown rice, wholewheat/gluten-free pasta, wholemeal/gluten-free bread, etc. Quality sources of protein are chicken, turkey, yoghurt, oily fish, tofu, peas, beans, nuts, seeds, etc.

Supplements can be included in the diet. It is preferable to get our vitamins and minerals from our food and the more unrefined food you eat, the greater the intake of vitamins and minerals. For example, wholewheat pasta and brown rice is packed full of B vitamins. Refined grains become white because the husk, which gives brown rice and wholewheat pasta its colour, has been stripped from it. This may make it look nice and white, but it actually takes all the vitamins and minerals out of it, leaving only a little bit of fibre. By eating lots of natural foods, such as fruit, vegetables, nuts, seeds, grains and pulses, you are going to be getting natural sources of your vitamins and minerals. For example, an avocado is loaded with vitamin E, whilst Brazil nuts are rich in selenium. However, we realise sometimes that you may want a little boost. If you wish to take a vitamin and mineral supplement, then it is okay to go ahead and do this. Always make sure that the supplement is within recommended daily amounts of each vitamin and mineral. Don't take any vitamin or mineral that has high levels, as these can be detrimental to your health in the long run. A good quality multivitamin is ideal. You don't need to take supplements every day, although this is perfectly fine if you follow the dosage label on supplement packaging. You may find that if you eat a very nutrient-dense diet, then you don't need a high dose of vitamins and minerals in supplement form. Many people use multivitamins as an insurance policy to ensure they meet the recommended intake of vitamins and minerals on a regular basis. This can be very useful for those with chronic health issues. Alternatively, you may wish to use vitamins and minerals when you specifically need them such as when you experience decreased immunity or have less energy. Vitamin C and zinc are particularly useful for treating and preventing cold and flu-type illnesses. Likewise, females may like to take a supplement containing B vitamins and magnesium at the "time of the month" to help relieve PMS symptoms and menstrual pain. B vitamins can additionally help to boost energy levels, whilst magnesium can also help to relieve pain and promote restful sleep. It has also become increasingly evident that low levels of vitamin D are common, so supplementing with this essential vitamin may be appropriate, especially during winter months. Taking vitamin and mineral supplements is not obligatory for good health. A healthy diet is far more important. However, a quality multivitamin does have its merits. Of course, if you have a known vitamin or mineral deficiency, then it is vital that you take the appropriate supplement to therapeutically treat this.

We particularly like probiotic supplements. Probiotics should contain lactobacillus acidophilus. It is even better if you are able to obtain supplements that have additional strains of probiotic present. The wider the range of probiotic strains, the greater the benefit. These are essential to replenish friendly bacteria within the gut. They benefit digestion and can improve immunity. Probiotics are found in fermented foods such as natural yoghurt, kefir, kombucha and miso. Taking a supplement can boost your intake further. Probiotics are essential for those with digestive problems and also if you suffer from chronic health issues, as the digestive tract plays a vital role in maintaining a healthy immune system. For this reason, almost everybody can benefit from taking them regularly, as a strong immune system is imperative to good health. When taking a probiotic, it is best to avoid eating or drinking hot food and/or beverages immediately afterwards, as the heat can destroy their beneficial properties. Also, look out for prebiotic supplements. These help to feed probiotics allowing good bacteria to survive and multiply in the gut. Prebiotics occur naturally in foods such as garlic, onions, chicory, bananas and yacon syrup. You can also take them in supplement form, many of which contain natural prebiotics such as inulin and Fructooligosaccharides (FOS). These can be beneficial when taken alongside a probiotic supplement.

An omega-3 supplement is also recommended. This is great for immunity, cardiovascular health and reducing inflammation. Again, eating regular portions of oily fish will boost the omega-3 content in your diet, but you can ensure good levels by taking a supplement on a daily basis. Omega oils can be found in fish oil, flaxseed oil and hemp seed supplements. Omega-3 fatty acids encourage the production of healthy prostaglandins that inhibit inflammation. There are different types of prostaglandins, those found in meats and cooking oils can cause inflammation, whereas good prostaglandins can actively prevent this. ALA, which can be found in flaxseed oil and walnuts, is converted into prostaglandins that provide beneficial results. Similarly, GLA is found in evening primrose oil and starflower oil. Supplements containing these oils are recommended for female health and are excellent for hormonal problems. Essential fatty acids are also great for skin problems, including eczema and dermatitis. If possible, opt for good quality, cold pressed varieties.

You may like to consider taking digestive enzymes if you experience any digestive problems or food intolerances. Enzymes help us to digest our food effectively. Whilst found in abundance in raw fruit and vegetables, supplementing with a plant-based digestive enzyme containing Betaine HCl can have a positive effect on digestive issues and may help to resolve such problems. Digestive enzymes help to break down food into molecules that are small enough to be absorbed within the digestive tract. If food is not broken down sufficiently, then we may not be able to absorb all the nutrients from our food. Undigested food can also pass into the lower gut and can begin to ferment due to the natural bacteria present. This can cause bloating, wind, indigestion and heartburn. Some people find that a digestive enzyme taken at the beginning of a meal can help them comfortably digest food and sufficiently ease symptoms, if this is usually a problem for them.

We also suggest including green superfoods such as barley grass in your diet. Barley grass is a great source of vitamins and minerals. It includes lots of B vitamins, is a good source of iron, vitamin C and vitamin K, which are all essential for good health. Barley grass is especially great if you buy it in powder form as this can be added to smoothies, salads, soups and yoghurts. It also has a great alkalizing effect on the body. As we discussed, it is preferable if the acid/alkaline balance is tipped in favour of the alkaline. Barley grass is great for providing an alkalizing intake into the diet. Spirulina, chlorella and wheatgrass are also good green alternatives. You may like to use green superfoods as an additional way of supplementing your diet instead of a multivitamin. You can also safely use this alongside vitamin and mineral supplementation. Green superfoods contain a lot of vitamins, minerals, essential amino acids and enzymes. However, as it is a natural food source, it can be harder to quantify exact amounts as you can do with multivitamins that have been formulated with recommended daily amounts. Additional supplements are not always necessary. However, green superfoods can complement and aid in the absorption of vitamin and mineral supplements. You can, of course, include lots of other superfood powders in your diet. For example, hemp is rich in protein and omega oils, whilst baobab is a good source of calcium and vitamin C. You can also add superfood powders to water and simply drink this. They can have a strong taste, so it is often more palatable to mix them into other drinks such as smoothies and juices. However, some do taste good this way. For example, baobab is nice mixed with cool water. Matcha, a type of green tea, is also a pleasant drink when mixed with warm or cool water.

Always buy good quality supplements, ensuring that you check the label if you have any food intolerances or allergies. There are a variety of supplements available that are free from gluten, dairy, lactose, sugar and yeast. Many supplements are made using gelatine. However, there are also many manufacturers who provide supplements suitable for vegetarians and vegans. Always follow the instructions on the supplement label. These will guide you on how often and the best way to take them. Unless otherwise stated, most supplements should usually be taken with a meal. This tends to be kinder on your stomach. Many vitamins and minerals are better absorbed when taken with food. If you have problems with your digestion, you may find softgel caps, liquid or spray formulas easier to take and less likely to irritate your tummy. Alternatively, if it is in tablet form you may like to halve this and take half in the morning and the other later in the day. Indeed, many people find this a useful way to take supplements, ensuring that their body efficiently absorbs the vitamins and minerals throughout the day as needed. Green superfood powders tend to be beneficial for those with weakened digestive systems. They are often better tolerated than supplements in tablet form. Each individual reacts differently and you should choose what works best for you.

Obviously, this information does not constitute medical advice. It is always advisable to consult your healthcare provider if you have any health concerns, wish to dramatically change your diet or include supplements. However, following a wholefood diet rich in fruit, vegetables, nuts, seeds and wholegrains will be nothing but beneficial.

We realise this can be a lot to take on board and can seem quite daunting, especially if there is a lot of new foods to be introduced. Most people panic when you suggest reducing sugar. However, once you begin to reduce your refined sugar intake, you will realise that you don't crave sugar as much. You will begin to enjoy the taste of fresh fruit and won't feel the need to eat a chocolate bar while you are watching television at night. Aim to change your diet over one to four weeks, depending on how good your diet is to begin with. Work at a rate that suits you. We want you to enjoy your new way of eating; following you will find a list of foods that are ideal to include in your diet. These are all available from good supermarkets and health food shops. You can often buy locally sourced and seasonal produce from regional butchers, fishmongers, greengrocers and farmer's markets. Try searching online for further quality wholefood suppliers.

Shopping List:

Where possible, buy organic. If applicable, choose raw, free-range, sustainably sourced and/or grass-fed/pastured varieties. Remember that the foods listed under sweeteners, sweets and snacks should be eaten in moderation. They should not be the main aspect of your diet. The focus of this should be on fruit, vegetables and wholefoods. Snacks, such as tortilla chips, are acceptable on occasion. Ensure that you opt for wholegrain varieties and serve with a healthy accompaniment such as houmous.

Fresh fruit: berries such as raspberries and blueberries, apples, lemons, limes, kiwis, avocados, bananas, grapes, oranges, etc.

Fresh vegetables: leafy green vegetables such as spinach and kale, carrots, sweet potatoes, peas, garlic, broccoli, cabbage, salad vegetables such as lettuce, cucumber, etc.

Pulses: red/green/brown lentils, split peas, beans, etc.

Grains: brown rice, spelt, millet, barley, quinoa, oats, amaranth, bulgur wheat, cornmeal, sprouted varieties, etc.

Breads: wholemeal, rye, spelt, corn, millet, quinoa, sourdough, gluten-free varieties, etc.

Flours: wholemeal, spelt, oat, soya, rice, gram, potato, buckwheat, almond, coconut, banana, sorghum, teff, tapioca, amaranth, etc.

Breakfast cereals: unsweetened/naturally sweetened muesli, granola, puffed rice, corn flakes, spelt flakes, and oat puffs, shredded wholewheat, oatmeal, quinoa flakes, rice flakes, grain-free varieties, etc.

Pastas: wholewheat, spelt, brown rice, quinoa, buckwheat, corn, lentil, other gluten/free pastas and noodles, etc.

Savoury biscuits: rice cakes, oatcakes, rye/spelt/gluten-free crackers and crispbreads, etc.

Spreads: houmous, tahini, coconut oil/butter, coconut jam, unsweetened fruit jam, unrefined nut butters such as almond, cashew, hazelnut, Brazil nut, peanut, etc.

Meat: beef, lamb, pork, venison, other lean game, etc.

Poultry: chicken, turkey, duck, goose, etc.

Fish: oily fish such as salmon, mackerel, tuna, trout, white fish such as cod, coley, haddock, seafood such as mussels, prawns, crab, etc.

Non-meat alternatives: Quorn, non-GMO tofu/soya/tempeh, etc.

Eggs: free-range hen eggs, duck eggs, goose eggs, quail eggs, etc.

Dairy: unsweetened natural/Greek yoghurt, cottage cheese, butter, ghee, cows'/ewes'/goats' milk and cheese, A2 milk, lactose-free milk and cheese, raw milk and cheese, etc.

Non-dairy: milks such as unsweetened/naturally sweetened rice, oat, soya, almond, cashew, hazelnut, coconut and hemp, dairy-free cheese and yoghurt, etc.

Freezer: vegetables such as edamame/broad/green beans, peas, spinach, corn, frozen fruit such as berries, etc.

Canned goods: vegetables with no added sugar/salt, tomatoes, chickpeas, beans, coconut milk, tinned fish, etc.

Stock: gluten/yeast/additive-free chicken and vegetable stock cubes, miso, vegetable bouillon, bone broth, etc.

Spices: cinnamon, cumin, ginger, chilli powder, cayenne, turmeric, coriander, curry, garam masala, Chinese 5 Spice, nutmeg, vanilla essence/powder, etc.

Seasoning: sea salt, herbal salt, pink Himalayan salt, whole black peppercorns, etc.

Condiments: tamari, Bragg Liquid Aminos, coconut aminos, raw apple cider vinegar, dairy/egg-free mayonnaise, nutritional yeast, unsweetened/naturally sweetened ketchup, etc.

Oils: extra virgin olive oil, rapeseed, coconut, sunflower, flaxseed, hemp seed, sesame, rice bran, red palm oil, etc.

Nuts: unsalted almonds, cashews, Brazil nuts, hazelnuts, macadamias, pine nuts, tiger nuts, etc.

Seeds: pumpkin, sesame, sunflower, hemp, chia, flaxseed, etc.

Superfood powders: barley grass, wheatgrass, spirulina, chlorella, hemp, baobab, lucuma, raw cacao, bee pollen, matcha, moringa, camu camu, maca, açai, pea protein, rice protein, ethically sourced gelatine/collagen, etc.

Fermented foods: milk kefir, water kefir, kombucha, sauerkraut, kimchi, etc.

Dried fruit: unsulphured apricots, figs, raisins, dates, goji berries, mulberries, etc.

Sweeteners: raw honey, agave nectar, xylitol, stevia, coconut sugar/nectar, rice malt/maple/yacon/carob/date syrup, Sweet Freedom, molasses, fruit sugar, raw cane sugar, etc.

Sweets: unsweetened/naturally sweetened cereal/seeded/nut-based bars, unsweetened/naturally sweetened carob, raw chocolate, raw cacao nibs, etc.

Snacks: unsweetened popcorn, vegetable/grain/pulse-based crisps, lightly salted/unsalted additive-free crisps and non-GMO corn tortillas, etc.

Beverages: water, herbal teas such as nettle, fennel, chamomile and peppermint, fruit teas such as raspberry, strawberry, apple and lemon, green tea, white tea, rooibos, barley/rye/dandelion/chicory coffee alternative, coconut water, fresh fruit/vegetable juice, naturally sweetened carbonated fruit juice, etc.

Sample menu:

So, what does a typical day of healthy eating look like then? Here are a few ideas that can be easily adapted to meet your dietary needs.

Breakfast: a bowl of porridge made with oats, water and/or non-dairy milk such as rice or almond milk. Serve with a handful of raspberries or grated apple and a sprinkling of sunflower seeds. A cup of hot water with a slice of unwaxed lemon and/or a glass of freshly squeezed vegetable juice.

Benefits: this is a healthy start to the day with the oats providing complex carbohydrates and fibre essential for healthy digestion. Gluten-free oats are available and suitable for gluten intolerance. Protein is added in the form of sunflower seeds and fruit provides one of your daily portions. For a grain-free version, you can have muesli made with fruit, coconut, nuts and seeds. The hot water and refreshing lemon has great detoxifying effects and is also good for digestion. Fresh juice provides an alkalising vegetable portion. Please don't skip this meal. If you really are not a breakfast person, try using the same ingredients in different quantities to make a smoothie. Blend some rice/almond milk with some fruit, along with a handful of oats and seeds, to make a filling drink. You can also add some protein-rich natural yoghurt or probiotic kefir with, or instead of, the sunflower seeds and, if you wish, omit the oats. Smoothies are also the ideal way to include superfood powders into your diet. You can easily add them in before you blend all your ingredients together.

Mid-morning snack: two rice cakes spread with houmous or almond nut butter. Serve with sliced cucumber sticks.

Benefits: this helps keep the body supplied with slow release energy to keep you going until lunch. Rice cakes made from brown rice are a good source of complex carbohydrates. Houmous provides some low-saturated fat and protein that also counts towards a vegetable portion, as does the alkaline-rich raw cucumber sticks. For a grain-free option, omit rice cakes and serve with additional fruit and/or vegetables.

Lunch: a bowl of vegetable soup with a sprinkling of toasted pumpkin seeds. Serve with a slice of wholemeal bread or two rye/gluten-free crispbreads with a small quantity of butter/dairy-free spread.

Benefits: the soup gives us another vegetable portion. Vegetable-based soups are a filling option and naturally lower in fat. Adding a handful of toasted seeds boosts the protein ratio and serving it with wholemeal bread or rye/gluten-free crispbreads provides a healthy portion of complex carbohydrates. You can easily substitute the bread for gluten-free options should you have a gluten intolerance. You can also omit the bread if you wish or if you are avoiding grains.

Mid-afternoon snack: two small kiwis and a small bowl of natural Greek yoghurt/a small avocado and/or a handful of raw, unsalted Brazil nuts or almonds/a natural fruit, nut and/or seed-based bar.

Benefits: the fruit provides another portion and the yoghurt is a good source of calcium and protein. Kiwis are rich in vitamin C, whilst avocado provides a serving of healthy fat. The nuts are a good source of protein and very rich in minerals. You can also have non-dairy yoghurt if you are avoiding all dairy produce. You may also prefer a healthy fruit, nut and/or seed-based bar as a little treat. This is especially good if you are on the go.

Evening meal: vegetable stir-fry made with onions, peppers, carrots, peas, courgettes. Top with chicken, salmon or tofu and serve with wholewheat/rice noodles or a few tablespoons of brown rice or quinoa. Finish with a few squares of raw chocolate.

Benefits: a stir-fry helps us meet our daily vegetable count. Chicken, salmon or tofu provides protein and the wholewheat/rice noodles, brown rice or quinoa provides slow release complex carbohydrates. If you are avoiding grains, you may omit these or try making vegetable-based noodles from courgettes or carrots using a spiralizer. A few squares of raw chocolate adds some low-fat, antioxidant-rich dairy and refined sugar-free sweetness. If you prefer, you can also try eating natural, unrefined bars made from fruit, nuts and seeds as a sweet treat.

Evening snack (optional): a small bowl of wholegrain cereal served with cows', rice, almond or hemp milk/two oatcakes thinly spread with lentil pâté. A cup of warm almond or rice milk. Top with grated nutmeg or half teaspoon each of ground turmeric, ginger, cinnamon and raw honey to taste.

Benefits: if you feel hungry or prefer to have a light supper, this will help you to nod off to sleep easily, thanks to the wholegrains, milk or lentils that contain the amino acid tryptophan known to help induce sleep. The wholegrain cereal and oats provides low-fat complex carbohydrates that will help to sustain blood sugar overnight. Opt for gluten-free varieties, if required. If you wish to avoid grains completely, you can substitute with small quantities of starchy complex carbs such as a small banana and a few nuts or seeds. A warm, milky drink is very soothing and can help promote a good night's sleep. Choose from any organic milk or non-dairy milk. Adding spices to the milk gives it an antioxidant boost. Nutmeg is a good source of copper and magnesium and a blend of turmeric, ginger and cinnamon provides anti-inflammatory properties. An evening snack should be higher in healthy carbohydrates and calcium, with medium to low levels of protein. Dairy, almond and hemp milk, nuts and pulses provide a small serving of protein. This should be a very small snack meal and should be eaten at least an hour before bedtime to prevent it from sitting too heavily in the stomach. Eating large meals too late at night can interfere with the digestive process and can cause discomfort, particularly in those with sensitive digestion.

Remember to drink plenty of healthy beverages throughout the day and voilà – you've just had a nutritious, wholefood day!

You will also find lots more clean eating recipes at the end of this book.

Lifestyle

Your choice of lifestyle habits greatly influences the quality of your life. Sleep and exercise, for example, are areas of great importance and giving these your attention can really boost how you feel.

Sleep is essential for health and wellbeing. It is our body's way of restoring and repairing. When we have adequate sleep, we tend to deal with stress more effectively. Establishing a regular sleep pattern is essential in maintaining wellbeing.

Try to go to bed at a regular time every night and arise around the same time each morning. This lets the body and mind know it is time for bed whilst also establishing a good sleeping pattern. If possible, at least 8 hours of sleep per day is ideal. However, an adult can function on anything between 6-10 hours sleep per day. As an individual, work out what is best for you.

Try to clear your mind as you are going to bed. Review the day, leaving any unfinished business for the next day. It may help to write down any thoughts that you have, perhaps any problems you have to solve or things you have to do, then leave them aside for tomorrow.

Avoid any stimulants before going to bed. This includes sugar, caffeine, cigarettes and alcohol. You want to induce a calm feeling in the body. Therefore, as previously discussed, a light snack or a warm drink is usually suffice. Similarly, avoid using the computer and other technology too close to bed as this keeps our minds active. The light transmitted from these is stimulating and you should try to switch off at least 1 hour before bed.

Ensure the bedroom is a pleasurable place to be. Keep clutter to a minimum. Make sure your bed is comfortable, your pillow is right and that the room is quiet and relaxed. You may like to try keeping your room dark whilst sleeping. This helps the body to produce the melatonin that helps you to sleep well. Blackout curtains and blinds can help, as does switching off all lights. Wearing a sleep mask, if you wish, can also be useful. Fresh air helps us get a better night's sleep, so open your window for a while every day to let air circulate around the room. Dehumidifiers can also help to keep the air fresh and reduce allergens in the room. Some people sleep better without distractions, such as television and radio, whilst other people particularly like to have music playing as they fall asleep. Obviously, always opt for relaxing music as opposed to loud, lively music which may keep you awake. If you like reading in bed, choose a book that you enjoy and that isn't too stimulating. You don't want to drift off into the land of nod having nightmares, so it may be best to avoid horror novels or hard-hitting stories from the newspaper. Instead, you might like to opt for inspiring or light-hearted reading material. Of course, please do what suits your individual tastes and whatever you personally find helps you relax and prepare for a good night's sleep.

You may wish to try putting a few drops of lavender essential oil on a tissue and place this by your pillow to help you drift off into a relaxed sleep. Try spritzing a lavender spray onto sheets and into the air to create a relaxing ambience. You can buy a good quality, natural lavender spray or simply make your own by adding around 12 drops lavender essential oil to 250ml water and store this in a spray bottle. Remember to give it a shake every time you use it to mix the oil and water together. Burning a lavender-infused candle can help induce relaxation. Opt for natural varieties and, for safety, always remember to extinguish before bedtime. Likewise, a bath can help us relax before bed. Make sure you don't have it immediately before going to bed as the hot water raises your body temperature. This can be too stimulating and prevent us from falling asleep right away. It is best to have your bath a couple of hours before bed, giving time for the body to cool down yet still allowing us to feel calm and relaxed. This warming and cooling action mimics the body's natural sleep rhythms. You can also add 6 to 8 drops of lavender essential oil to your bath water. Similarly, bath oils containing lavender are good to use too. This will not only condition your skin but also help to create a relaxing atmosphere as you inhale the lavender. This helps you to fall asleep more easily. You might like to rub a little lavender essential oil onto your temples or wrists to help you to relax and promote restful sleep. You can also buy good quality sleep balms, made from natural ingredients, which commonly contain lavender essential oil to help you relax. Applying a hand or foot cream, made using lavender essential oil, is useful too as the calming properties can help to soothe. Essential oils are absorbed by the skin. Applying a cream made with lavender can have a sleep inducing effect. Try, where possible, to choose a cream free from parabens and synthetic ingredients. These can have carcinogenic properties and a detrimental effect on the hormonal system. The skin is our largest organ and we absorb whatever we put on it, so opt instead for a natural formulation. Now, if you have a favourite cosmetic product that isn't natural you don't need to throw it away, especially if it makes you feel good when using it. Common sense should be applied. In order to be legally sold, a product has been certified as safe to use. However, we would recommend that you limit the use of products that have chemical ingredients and make the majority of your cosmetic regime as natural as possible. In addition to parabens, limit the use of products containing phthalates and aluminium. These are also thought to have carcinogenic properties. Parabens and phthalates, in particular, have been found to be endocrine disrupters that can adversely affect hormones. Toxins, known as xenoestrogens, can be found in cosmetics as well as pesticides, plastics and household chemicals. These can disrupt the endocrine system by mimicking hormones in the body. You don't need to be obsessive about this, but reducing your exposure to these toxins will be beneficial to your hormonal system and your general health. Err on the side of caution when it comes to artificial ingredients and preservatives.

Regular exercise can help us to experience deeper and more restful sleep. Be sure to perform any exercise 2-4 hours before sleeping so that you don't stimulate the body too much. Choose what exercise suits you best and what would be most appropriate for inducing sleep. If you do choose to exercise before bed, make sure it is a relaxing form that helps you to de-stress and not invigorate you too much. For example, ideal exercises are gentle stretching, Pilates, yoga and Tai Chi.

When falling asleep, it may help to visualise a pleasant scene or thought in your mind. This helps to quieten the mind and relax us. If you wake up during the night, try repeating a word to help you fall back to sleep. Repeating a word, such as "sleep" or "relax", can help us get back into sleep mode.

If you do find that you cannot sleep, it can be useful to get up. The worst thing you can do is to stay in bed and brood over any problems. It may be helpful to get up, perhaps read a book or have a cup of herbal tea that will help to induce sleep. Then once you feel sleepy again, return to bed and this should help you to fall over to sleep more easily. Herbal teas, such as chamomile and valerian, can help promote sleep. As they are free from caffeine, they don't have a stimulating effect. You can also buy a selection of teas made with a blend of herbs that specifically aid sleep. If your sleep pattern is problematic, you might like to keep a few of these herbal teas to hand to drink as required. You may wish to start a nightly routine of making your evening drink a soothing herbal tea.

Some people can have problems with their sleep pattern. Quality sleep can be an issue for many people and particularly for those with insomnia and/or chronic health problems. If our sleep is disturbed, it can increase fatigue levels and cause our muscles to become sore due to the lack of adequate rest. Developing good sleep hygiene is necessary. Poor sleep obviously makes us feel more tired and if you already have health problems, this can cause a flare-up in symptoms. Make sleep a priority in your life. Realise that it plays an important part of our overall wellbeing. We need to have a good sleep pattern in order to keep us refreshed and revitalised. Should your sleep be interrupted, take it easy and try to have an early night the next day to help your body replenish. Hopefully, as you incorporate the advice given, you will see the quality of your sleep improve.

Sleep is the ultimate relaxation. Just as it is vital to look after your diet, the management of sleep habits is an important lifestyle factor for keeping stress at a minimum and wellbeing at a maximum. Go ahead, relax and catch some zzzz's.

Our bodies are also designed to be physically active on a regular basis. This helps to manage stress and promote health and wellbeing.

It is easy in today's lifestyle to become sedentary. This can have ill effects on our health. For example, a lifestyle lacking adequate exercise can lead to heart disease and obesity. By exercising regularly, you can help to strengthen your heart and prevent the build-up of fatty deposits on the artery wall. Therefore, the more you exercise, the healthier you become and you will have more energy for other activities. If your body is fit, it can handle more. Your body will become more efficient in using up calories, doesn't tire so quickly and muscles become stronger, which helps you to manage stress far better and helps you sleep more effectively.

There are many types of exercise that you can choose. Make sure that you enjoy the form of exercise that you opt for. Otherwise, it becomes too easy to give into the temptation to abandon your new fitness regime. Perhaps some of the most relaxing exercises to do are yoga, Pilates and Tai Chi. This is a fantastic way of relieving stress, improving posture and fitness levels as well as calming the mind. Exercise, such as yoga, works not only to release tension but also psychologically as you focus on specific slow movements allowing the mind to open. This can help create balance and initiate healing. Exercise releases endorphins, a natural hormone, which helps to relieve stress and boost the feeling of wellbeing. You should try to incorporate some aerobic exercise into your fitness regime to help further control stress. Holding on to stress and tension can lead to exhaustion and muscle pain. Aerobic exercise does not have to be something vigorous. Walking, cycling and swimming are ideal and economical ways to burn off extra calories, promote better sleep, provide an ideal time to think and help get rid of excess stress.

You should aim to exercise regularly. We must learn to recognise what works best for our body. You can then implement this gradually. Aim to get some form of exercise every day. Remember that short bursts of exercise are better than lengthy yet sporadic activity. For example, start by walking 5-10 minutes every day, then build up and increase the length of time you walk by 5 minutes per day until you are walking for at least 30 minutes, at least three times a week. Try to select interesting walks and avoid busy areas where fuel fumes tend to accumulate. If you can walk to work or the local bus/train station, then try this. It is an excellent way to increase our physical activity and endorphins, the body's happy hormones, are released helping us to feel good.

We realise that we all have different health and energy levels. For example, if you suffer from health issues, such as limited or reduced mobility, extreme fatigue and pain, then the last thing you want to do is exercise. Even if you would like to, often your body is just too exhausted and sore to make the effort. Exercise can be of great help to those who have a chronic condition. It can help to boost energy levels, relieve pain and improve our sleep quality. It is all about finding the right balance. Start by introducing gentle exercise at a level that suits you. If you can only manage 5 minutes, then that is fine. A gentle walk for 5-10 minutes or a few simple yoga poses can make all the difference. Pace yourself, ensuring that you do not push yourself too far. You should start off slow, aiming to do what you feel you comfortably can within your limits, working up to around 30 minutes exercise approximately three times per week. It's great if you can do this but just as good if you can only manage a few minutes when you feel able. Work at your own level. You want to energise not exhaust yourself. Through time, you will notice that you feel better. You might feel less tired, more flexible or notice that you are not quite as sore. As your symptoms improve and become more manageable, you may be able to increase your activity level. Please remember to always respect your body. Take rest days and work at your own pace.

Should you choose to undertake energetic exercise, such as aerobics or endurance sports, you might like to consider what you eat and drink both before and after the physical activity. Eat a snack around 30-40 minutes prior to exercising. Try combining complex carbohydrates with a healthy protein. Complex carbohydrates are easily digested and help to raise energy levels, whilst protein can help muscles recover from exertion. For example, you can eat wholegrain bread with almond butter or natural Greek yoghurt with a chopped banana. You might also like to snack on a mixture of fruit, nuts and seeds. You can find a recipe for this later in the book. Following your workout, ensure you restore your energy levels within 20-60 minutes by eating protein with complex carbohydrates. Eating within this timeframe helps muscle recovery and replenishes the body's glycogen stores. An omelette made with lots of fresh vegetables or a baked sweet potato topped with tahini are good examples of healthy post-workout meals. Of course, if you don't have time or if it simply isn't convenient to prepare a meal before or after exercise, you can always have a ready-made protein bar or shake. Avoid products made with unwanted additives. Look for those made with natural ingredients or make your own instead. A smoothie made with fresh fruit, nut milk and a natural protein powder, such as hemp, is much healthier than some of the commercial sports drinks available. Ensure that you stay hydrated and drink lots of water. Make sure you drink plenty throughout the day. Don't just overload on water right before your workout. This will not hydrate you instantly. It may even cause you to feel uncomfortable during exercise. Avoid caffeinated sports drinks. These are usually full of sugar or artificial sweeteners and colourants. Stick to water or try drinking coconut water, which has naturally occurring potassium and electrolytes that help you stay hydrated. If you are not doing excessively strenuous exercise, you don't need to worry too much about what you eat and drink before and after working out. However, it is always best to avoid exercising on a full stomach, regardless of the activity level, in order to ensure your comfort. Always remember to keep water to hand too.

Most importantly, choose a form of exercise you like and look forward to doing. There are lots of ways that you can incorporate regular exercise into your life. For example, you can join a class, workout alone or use an exercise DVD/online video at home. Do what feels best for you and remember to enjoy it. Now, there's no excuse. Let's get moving.

Relaxation

It is important to make time to relax. Relaxation is vital to health and wellbeing. Everybody needs to make time to rest. Think how tired you can feel after a busy day. Taking time to relax helps to replenish our energy levels. Not allowing yourself to relax can lead to excessive stress and subsequent ill health.

But, honestly, how many of us truly make the time to relax properly? Grabbing a cup of coffee and slouching in front of the television isn't relaxing; neither is dozing off for 5 minutes on the couch. To truly unwind, we have to make the effort to consciously relax. By consciously relaxing, we bring our awareness into the present moment. As we begin to focus our mind, we find that we become calmer, our breathing slows down and we react less to stressful situations. Relaxation also helps us to feel more serene, less tense and more creative.

It is best to find a quiet place to practice relaxation where you will not be interrupted for at least 15 minutes. Lying down comfortably, sitting on a cushion or a well-backed chair ensures that the spine is straight and the body still. Hands should be at your side with palms facing upwards, if lying down. Otherwise, they should rest lightly on your thighs, palm side up. Turning your hands to face upwards helps to rotate and open the shoulders. You can do this in silence or, if you prefer, you can play some relaxing instrumental music in the background. You may wish to put on some extra clothing such as a cardigan or jumper. Alternatively, you can cover yourself with a blanket because your body's metabolism will be slowing down and, as a result, you may feel cooler.

Try to establish a time that you will set aside for relaxation. Do what is best for you. Perhaps you would like to practice every morning or evening, possibly even both. Ensure you make time. Don't automatically assume you don't have time. If you can make time to watch television, read the newspaper or constantly worry, then you can find time for relaxation. It is great if you can dedicate 15 minutes or more once or twice a day. However, if you can only manage 5 minutes per day, then this is good too. The key is to practice a relaxation technique regularly, ideally every day. You will instantly feel calmer and, over time, you will notice that you cope better with stress, have more energy and generally feel better in both body and mind.

Following you will find examples of relaxation techniques. All of them are useful and work equally well. Try each of the exercises and see what you most enjoy. You can choose just one to do every day or you can vary exercises so that you don't get bored. As long as you make time to relax, you can't go wrong.

Each exercise is simple to undertake. Keeping it simple makes it easier to remember and after practicing these a few times you will soon be able to do it without reading the instructions, as you will easily be able to recall them. If you prefer to listen to the relaxation exercises, you can record yourself reciting them. If you do not like listening to your own voice, you can ask someone else to record them so that you can simply listen as you go along. There is also a wide range of relaxation exercises available in formats such as CD, MP3, apps and online video. You can also use these if you wish to add some variety.

Progressive muscle relaxation is where we consciously tense the muscles and then relax them. Just as the body has the ability to go into fight or flight response, making us ready for action, we can also influence our body to reach a state of relaxation. The following exercise encourages us to relax using simple techniques.

Lie on the floor with your legs straight out. If that strains your back, either bend them at the knees or sit comfortably on a chair. Your arms should be relaxed, about three to four inches away from your side. Feel the floor or chair supporting your body. Feel the heaviness of the body. Notice your breath, imagine you can see it entering and leaving the nostrils. Breathe normally, but be aware of this. Beginning at the toes, consciously relax each part of the body in turn. You can tense each part and then relax it. Alternatively, you may find it easier to imagine that specific part of the body relaxing. So, relax the right foot, the right calf, the right thigh, the left foot, the left calf, the left thigh, relax the buttocks, the abdomen, the rib cage and the chest. Relax the muscles in the back and relax the spine. Relax the right shoulder, the right upper arm, the right forearm and the right hand. Relax the left shoulder, the left upper arm, the left forearm and the left hand. Relax the front of the neck and the back of the neck. Relax the jaw and relax the cheeks. Relax the area around the eyes and the area between the eyebrows. Relax the forehead and relax the scalp. Check over your body for any tension and release any that you find. Think of the body relaxing and the mind relaxing. Imagine all the tension draining from the body. Notice your breath. See it as it enters and leaves the nostrils. As you breathe out, tell yourself that it is carrying away all the tension and negative, stressful feelings. Continue this for at least 5 minutes. Once you are ready, bring your awareness back to your breathing and gently open your eyes. Take your time to come back to reality and when you are ready, slowly sit up.

Through physically relaxing, we can learn to relax our mind as well as our body. This helps us to release our need to always be in control. As we free our muscles from tension, we can free our mind from anxiety and stress. This can boost our immune system and give us a sense of immense wellbeing.

The following exercise is a combination of breathing techniques and meditation. When we become stressed, our breathing becomes more rapid and shallow. There is a link between breathing and relaxation. If we consciously alter our breathing pattern, then we can slow down our breathing rate and induce relaxation. Meditation is a way of relaxing and focusing on the mind. This exercise is simple and effective. It can be used regularly for deep relaxation.

Sit or lie down in a comfortable position and close your eyes. Take a deep breath and hunch your shoulders. Lift them up to your ears and hold them tight. Hold your breath for a few seconds. This should never be uncomfortable. Breathe out slowly and, as you do, allow your shoulders and jaw to relax. Let your arms become limp.

Then carry on breathing normally. Breathe in and as you breathe out start counting down from ten. Breathe in again and on the next exhalation count nine and so forth until you reach one. You can then say the number one repeatedly, you can start to count backwards from ten again or you can simply let your mind wander. Continue this for approximately 3-20 minutes.

If any unwanted thoughts or worries begin to creep in, just simply let them be. Let them drift off and do not put too much focus on them. This will inevitably happen when you first start to practice relaxation. The more regularly you practice, the less this will begin to happen. It may help to start counting back from ten again or just to repeat the number one to help refocus your mind and distract it from any unwanted thoughts. Some people prefer to repeat a certain word such as "still", "peace" or "calm". Any word that really helps you to relax. If you wish to repeat this word once you have reached number one, feel free to do so. This can also be used if you feel unwanted thoughts creep in while relaxing to help you refocus. Simply repeat your chosen word until your mind becomes still again. Of course, you don't need to repeat any words. You can simply relax and rest in the silence. Once the exercise is complete, open your eyes slowly and focus on an object around you in the room in order to bring your awareness back to normal day activities. Then go about the rest of your day feeling relaxed and calm.

Visualisation encourages us to relax by imagining ourselves involved in a peaceful situation. Through this imagery, we are able to relax and calm the body and mind. There are many techniques we can use for visualisation. It may be that you take an imaginary journey, thinking of yourself floating on a cloud, gently moving downstream or resting by a warm fire. As long as you can daydream, there is no reason you can't visualise and promote relaxation.

There is no wrong way to visualise. As long as you imagine yourself in the visualisation, then you are encouraging the body to relax. The following visualisation involves us going on an imaginary journey onto a beach. However, if you don't feel that this works for you, by all means change it to a colourful garden, a freshly cut meadow or whatever you feel works best for you.

Get yourself comfortable, lie or sit as we've discussed before, and gently close your eyes. Imagine yourself lying on warm, golden sand. Feel the warmth of the sun radiating over your body. Hear the peaceful lapping of waves and the soothing song of distant birds. Feel the warm, gentle breeze upon your skin and take a deep breath, inhaling the clean, pure air. As you exhale, feel yourself sink deeper into the warm, soft sand. Relax with every breath, gently basking in the sunlight and sand. As you do this, imagine all the stress and tension flow away with every exhalation as you let go. The more you do this visualisation, the more you become a part of the scene. You may imagine yourself relaxing as you lie on the sand with the warm sun beating down on you.

You may eventually find that when you are in a stressful situation all you need to do is conjure up the image of your visualisation. For example, if you are under extreme pressure and feeling very tense, perhaps all you will need to do is close your eyes and see yourself lying on that warm beach basking in the sun. This will instantly produce a feeling of relaxation, calm and wellbeing.

We realise, at times, you may encounter stress when it is not possible to do relaxation exercises. By regularly doing the exercises described, you will find that you cope better with stress and have increased wellbeing. Your immune system is also boosted and overall you will feel the benefit of doing this on a regular basis. However, if you encounter stress within daily life, there are some instant relaxation techniques that can help you to cope with that stress as it happens. These also help to stop you reacting negatively to stress.

There are some easy ways to distract our body from stress throughout the day. If you find yourself stressed, for example at work, where possible stop the stressful activity and remove yourself from the situation in order to give you time to recollect. Going for a short walk, if possible, is useful in helping you clear your mind. A short, brisk walk can help to release muscle tension, allowing for the flow of oxygen around the body as well as providing a mental diversion. You can use this time to think positive thoughts or repeat any affirmations to yourself that will help break that stress cycle. Walking also provides time to think. Don't think deliberately, allow yourself time to process any problems. You may find that solutions spring to mind more easily whilst walking.

Taking one or two slow, deep breaths can help to rebalance breathing and calm the body and mind. This is a quick and simple technique that brings about a relaxation response, which can be done throughout the day, whether there is a stressful situation or not. When you take your one or two deep breaths, try to push your stomach out as you take the breath. If possible, hold this for 2-3 seconds and then exhale with a long, slow breath. As you exhale, let your shoulders and jaw drop. You should feel the relaxation flow from your neck and shoulders, down your arms to the fingertips. This is very effective in correcting shallow breathing whilst releasing the tension that most of us carry in our neck and shoulders.

Another simple way of reducing stress is to write down how you are feeling or, indeed, write anything in order to distract yourself from that stressful situation. Picking up a pen or pencil and doodling away can help just as well. Colouring books, including adult varieties, are widely available. These can divert our attention from current problems and demands, helping us to become more mindful as we focus on the process of colouring in the picture. A simple action, such as splashing your face or wrists with cool water, can also help to distract you and to calm your body when under stress. Many people find that prayer provides an opportunity to relax, communicate and share our problems with our higher power, creator or whatever your spiritual alignment may be.

Stretching is a good way to focus on relaxing muscles quickly and consciously. Try to stretch as far as you possibly can by attempting to reach the ceiling with both hands. Make sure your weight is balanced evenly between both feet, which should be hip width apart. Try putting both your arms behind your back, at hip level, then clasp your hands and pull down your back. This will open your chest and shoulders. If you feel like it, you can yawn and then relax your arms completely by your side.

Music can also help us to relax. Choosing soft and relaxing music to play in the background can help us to feel more calm and relaxed. Similarly, music can provide a distraction if you are feeling very stressed. In this situation, you can use music to distract you from these feelings. It doesn't necessarily have to be relaxing music. Any music that you enjoy, which can take your mind off problems, can help make us feel more calm and able to cope better. However, listening to relaxing music helps to create an inner calm that can be useful, for example, when we are commuting. Although there might be a lot of activity going on around you, relaxing music can help us to stay serene whilst the surrounding environment is filled with movement. Listening to music whilst exercising, such as walking, is another great way to relax. Choose a tempo that suits your pace. Let it help focus and relax your mind as you enjoy your walk.

Dance, like music, can also help us to relax. You don't need to have followed dance as a discipline, just allow yourself to be led by the music. In doing so, dancing can deeply relax the body and mind. The best way to do this is to simply put on some music and dance around the house, for example, whilst you are cleaning. If you feel conscious of doing this, do so when you know you will not be interrupted and no one else is around. Alternatively, you may wish to join a dance class. Dance allows us to let go of any tension in the body. It is good for boosting the heart rate and giving us a short burst of exercise. It also, again, helps to distract us from any feelings that may be making us tense and wound up, helping to relax the body and mind. Dancing helps us to use up energy, making us feel happier whilst giving our wellbeing a boost.

Massage is another powerful way to bring about relaxation. It is very comforting and improves our wellbeing. It helps to relax aching muscles and reduce stress levels. It also helps lower blood pressure, relieve pain, strengthen the immune system, improve circulation and increase our energy levels. If you can have a professional massage; then this is great. Massages are a wonderful way of relaxing our muscles and, in doing so, we get used to being in a more relaxed state in both body and mind. Like with all other relaxation techniques, when stress does occur we tend to deal with it a lot better when we become used to feeling relaxed on a regular basis.

We can also perform self-massage. This might not be as thorough as a half-hour professional back massage, but it can still help us to relax and by doing it ourselves, there is no reason why we can't do it as often as we wish. This can be every day, once a week or whenever you feel tense. By regularly doing this, you will feel the benefits. One of the simplest techniques is to massage your scalp. When you are tense, the skin on your scalp doesn't move easily on the skull beneath. Sit as relaxed as you can in a comfortable chair. Starting above the forehead, using the fingers of both hands, trace small circular strokes. Using a light to medium pressure, work slowly backwards on either side towards the top of your neck, then outwards behind your ears and up and out at the temples. If you think of the technique you use to massage shampoo into your hair as you wash it; then this is a similar movement. Simply just massaging the head can help to loosen any tightness that is present in the scalp and help us to relax. Although working only on the head, it has an overall effect on the body, helping us to calm down and breathe more easily.

We also carry a lot of tension in our eyes, which is not something we necessarily think of. We tend to think of carrying tension in the neck, which we do, but our eyes are also constantly in use. They come under a lot of strain from not only computers and overhead lighting, but in general, when we are tired and stressed causing a lot of tension in the facial area. So, gently rub your hands together to build up a little bit of friction and heat. Place your palms, one over each eye. You will feel a gentle warmth. This will help to relax the eye area and any tension whilst helping us to relax overall. As you are doing this, it can be useful to take a couple of deep breaths, just to further that relaxation response.

Another great self-massage technique is to work over the neck. The neck obviously carries a lot of tension. We can get a lot of pain in our neck just through everyday movements due to the fact that most of us have quite a sedentary lifestyle now. Before massaging the neck, it is advisable to remove any jewellery present. Sit in a comfortable chair and relax your neck and shoulders as much as you can. Then using the fingers of both hands stroke either side of the neck, avoiding the spinal area. Use a light pressure at first, building up to a more firm pressure, stroke up towards the skull and then down again. Then you can begin to knead the same area lightly again, building up to a more firm pressure. You can continue this movement onto the shoulders, sitting in the same position. Use your right hand for the left shoulder and left hand for the right shoulder. Just pick up and squeeze the muscles that cover the shoulder. Start from the neck and work towards the edge of the shoulder. Pick this up, gently squeeze and then let go. This helps to resolve any tension we are carrying in the shoulder area.

You don't have to use any oil with self-massage. However, you can buy a pre-blended massage oil or use a carrier oil, such as sweet almond oil or olive oil, and add a few drops of lavender essential oil. In doing so, whilst massaging, you will inhale the essential oils. This has a relaxing effect. Also, as you apply the oil onto your skin, the body absorbs this into the bloodstream giving a further relaxing effect. Unless you are a qualified aromatherapist, you are not advised to blend a lot of essential oils for safety reasons. However, it is quite safe to use lavender oil. In fact, lavender essential oil, also known as Lavandula Angustifolia, can be used neat and is always a handy oil to have around for first aid purposes as this can be applied straight to burns to soothe any irritation. Some people can be sensitive to essential oils, so use what is best for you. If you are pregnant, essential oils can occasionally cause problems. Whilst lavender is generally okay to use, it is advisable to avoid using it on the skin in the first trimester of pregnancy. If you do choose to blend your own oil, you should use about 15ml of oil and into this add 1 or 2 drops of lavender essential oil. This is all you will need, as essential oils are very potent and this is enough for personal use. If you prefer a stronger oil, you can add up to 5 drops essential oil. You can apply this to the scalp, if you wish, during massage. By leaving this on you not only provide a relaxing treatment but the oils will also penetrate and have a conditioning effect on skin and hair. You can use this oil as a therapeutic body oil that can be applied to skin after a shower or bath. You can also use it as a skin cleanser, facial oil and/or moisturiser, taking care to avoid the delicate eye area. You might also like to try making this oil with coconut oil, which although solid at room temperature, melts easily upon contact with the skin. This has great skin and hair care properties. Essential oils and base oils are best purchased from an aromatherapy supplier or reputable outlet to ensure that you get good quality oils. Opt for unrefined, therapeutic grade and, where possible, organic varieties.

In addition to essential oils, you may find it helpful to use semi-precious gemstone crystals as these are believed to assist in healing and can help benefit body and mind. Some crystals, such as rose quartz and amethyst, are said to have relaxation properties. Rose quartz is believed to promote love, help release anger and aid sleep, whilst amethyst is thought to be a meditative and calming stone that promotes balance and peace. You can simply carry a piece of the gemstone with you, tuck it under your pillow or wear gemstone jewellery. You can also have a professional crystal healing treatment/massage. During this, a therapist will place specific crystals on strategic areas. Remember other complementary therapies, such as reflexology, reiki, osteopathy and magnet therapy, can be very beneficial too. Choose therapies that work for you. Opt for those that you feel comfortable with and that encourages you to relax.

We should also remember that our hobbies and interests count as relaxation as we tend to relax when we do something we enjoy. For example, gardening is a very relaxing pastime. Not only does it help us to physically burn off excess energy, which is useful after a stressful day, but it also helps us to get rid of tension and frustration. It also has meditative qualities as you connect with nature. Combined with fresh air, it helps to boost our mood as well as improving vitamin levels, thanks to natural source Vitamin D from sunlight.

Hobbies, such as crafts like knitting and sewing, are also very relaxing as they have a meditative effect. The repetition of knitting, stitching or following a pattern allows us to focus our minds onto what we are doing. As we do this, we become very much in the present moment. Therefore, crafts are very similar to meditation. They help us create mindfulness where we are focused on what we are doing. If you are a crafter, you can use this time to focus on how you are feeling. As you get lost in that repetitive motion, you will notice that many problems that are bothering us have a tendency to slip away. We find that when we focus on the present, sometimes solutions to problems we have been worrying about just suddenly come to us or problems don't seem quite so bad. As well as being creative, they have a very relaxing effect. When we feel we are being creative, we tend to feel more relaxed and more inspired and, in turn, our wellbeing is boosted.

Reading is another hobby that is a good way of relaxing. Reading a funny or calming book helps to take your mind off situations and problems as you can literally lose yourself in a book. Of course, you can choose any genre of book that you enjoy reading. Problems that trouble us in everyday life don't seem so bad whilst reading a book, as we distract ourselves from what is happening around us. By focusing visually on the words, we focus less on other things.

As well as using relaxation exercises, we can also use our everyday hobbies to cope with stress more effectively.

Incorporating these relaxation exercises into our daily lives, particularly through progressive muscle relaxation, breathing meditation and visualisation, can really have a powerful effect on our health and wellbeing. Implementing the instant stress relievers, such as taking a walk or having a good stretch, are great ways to keep us refreshed throughout the day. Even better if you can also add in massage techniques, be it professional or self-massage. All of these things introduced on a regular basis have an overall effect on our wellbeing. Regular relaxation will help us to cope more effectively with stress. You will find that the more often you do this, you will notice that your muscles become less tense, your breathing is more calm and efficient whilst your immune system and overall health and wellbeing receive a boost.

Calm down and relax, it's good for you!

Positive Thinking

A positive attitude can help us to not only create wellbeing but also boost our immune system and change our outlook for the better. While we know that feeling positive won't miraculously make all your problems disappear, it can certainly help us to feel better about ourselves and our situation. A positive attitude helps us cope better with stress, ill health and life in general. Adopting a happy, positive demeanour can really help and all you have to do is learn some simple techniques.

Our mind is comprised of the conscious and the subconscious. The conscious mind is rational and helps us to make decisions on a daily basis, while the subconscious mind deals with behaviour that we have already learned and stores information should we need it again. For example, this is useful when we learn to ride a bike. The subconscious mind stores it so we don't have to consciously find our balance every time. However, the subconscious mind is highly suggestible. It can't process wrong from right, it simply stores information that we can use once again later. It is the same with our thoughts. If you constantly think that you are not good enough or don't believe in yourself, then the subconscious mind believes this too. Therefore, it stands to reason that if we can convince our subconscious mind into believing negative statements, then we can also make it believe positive ones.

Instead of thinking, for example, "things always go wrong" think "things will go right". Instead of thinking, "I feel bad about myself" think "I feel good about myself". Instead of thinking, "I am in pain" think "I will feel better". In doing so, you are not denying how you are feeling, but you are adopting a positive attitude that can help you to improve your mind. A positive outlook can help us to initiate healing within the body.

Notice the words you use when speaking. Perhaps you have a habit of putting yourself down. If you do, now is the time to stop it and give yourself a bit of respect. Have love and compassion for yourself, despite your faults. We are all human and none of us is perfect. Think about how many times you say the word "can't" such as "I can't do this", "I can't do that" or "yes, I'd like to, but I can't". Try to adjust your outlook. A great way of doing this is to simply strike off the "t" in the word "can't", this then becomes "can". Instead of saying "I can't do it", you now say "I can do it". Striking off the "t" helps turn negative phrases into positive statements. For every negative thing you say or do, try to replace this with a positive.

A lot of us have the tendency to complain more than we should do. It is easy to focus on things that aren't right, but instead, try to concentrate on the good stuff. At the end of the day, think about what you can be grateful for in your life. By switching from a state of complaining to that of being thankful, you can lift your mood, especially during low moments. Over time, by doing this regularly, you will notice that you become aware of and appreciate good things happening to you.

Similarly, say "thank you" regularly throughout the day. Try this when you wake in the morning to help start your day on a positive thought. Try to notice things you can be thankful for. They can be little things from being thankful for enjoying a nice cup of tea to being appreciative of a special person. Develop an attitude of gratitude for a positive outlook. The more you do it, the more you attract and notice things to be thankful for.

Learn to recognise your positive qualities. It is too easy to focus on the things you think you can't do and other negative thoughts. Try instead to identify positive aspects. Think about yourself and write down any of your positive traits such as patience, good humour, friendliness, etc. Once you have written down your positive traits, you may like to keep your list nearby so that if you feel negative about yourself, you can have a quick look at this to remind you of your positive attributes.

Likewise, you may want to think about what you have done recently. List any positive things you have undertaken. At first, you may not be able to think of anything, but if you think over all the tasks you have completed, you are sure to find something positive. This could be something as simple as being organised enough to clean out a cluttered cupboard, having learned how to use new computer software at work or taking the initiative to have enrolled in an exercise class. Give yourself credit for any effort, success and achievements, no matter how big or small.

Keeping a record of our positive thoughts helps us to feel better about ourselves, creating more positivity in our lives. Not only do we feel good about ourselves when we keep a note of all the good things in our life, it can also help us to notice good things about other people and life in general.

You might like to consider keeping a "positivity journal". How do we do this? All you need to do is write down what you're thankful for and keep note of positive things you notice in your life. Research has shown that when we actively look for things to be grateful about, then we actually become happier and more content with our life. As a positive attitude is essential to your overall wellbeing, we think it is worthwhile taking time to keep a positivity journal. Try to do this daily. Simply write down at least one thing that you are thankful for and one positive thing you've noticed. We are sure that you will feel more positive and upbeat. As you do this regularly, you will find lots to be thankful and positive about. You will easily be able to write more things down. Pick a time each day to set aside to complete your positivity journal. It will only take a few minutes, but you will undoubtedly reap the benefits for such a small investment of your time. You might find it useful to fill in your journal in the evening when you can review your day and think about what good things happened. Dedicating time to positive thoughts in the evening can also put us in a relaxed, happy state of mind and helps to induce restful sleep.

You may like to use a notebook to create your journal. Use this to record your thoughts and feelings. Choose an attractive notebook that is a pleasure to write in and that you enjoy looking at. Make it as pleasurable as possible so that you enjoy writing in it. You might also like to create and print out a page with space for you to write all your positive thoughts. You can then keep the pages in a folder and create your positivity journal. Again, choose a nice ring binder or suitable folder.

Personalise your journal, customise it to make it your own. For example, you don't have to stick to using a blue or black pen. Try using different colour pens or pencils. You can also decorate it with doodles and photographs that mean something to you. Of course, you can keep it simple by just writing down your positive thoughts. Do what feels best for you, but most importantly, use it regularly. We promise you will feel better in doing so.

Now, we realise that we don't always have fantastic lives and that sometimes things don't go to plan. However, keeping a positivity journal helps us to focus on the positive aspects of our lives. By taking time to think positively, we start to notice that we actually attract more happy and positive things into our lives. Also, if you should happen to have an off day, simply read what you have written previously to help focus on the good things that you have or has already happened to you. It doesn't need to be all-singing, all-dancing things to make it worth writing in our journal. Simple things, such as family, friends, nice things people did for you or you did for them, good weather, good food, personal attributes and achievements, are all positive things you can write down. It doesn't matter if you write similar things each day, just make the effort and you will definitely start to notice more things to be thankful and positive about.

Developing a positive attitude can help us cope better with whatever life throws at us. A happy and content outlook can help us achieve wellbeing and creates balance in our lives. If any problems do arise, learn to accept them and realise that this can happen as part of life. Acknowledge it, take action if appropriate, but don't let your problems rule you. We know it can be difficult at times but think positive and be grateful. Love yourself and love your life, no matter how challenging. Stay positive and you will begin to feel better in both body and mind.

Consider your body language. Take a look at your posture; a lot of us have the tendency to slouch with our shoulders hunched and our head jutting forward. Not only does this cause strain on our muscles, but it can also make us look downtrodden and make us feel bad about ourselves. It can help us to look and feel better if we stand up straight and relax our shoulders, pushing them down, round and back whilst tucking our chin inwards. Try imagining that you have a balloon tied to your head pulling it upwards. By becoming aware of our posture, we help to give ourselves a boost physically and mentally.

Likewise, try to laugh and smile more. We use more muscles to frown. Smiling makes us look better, feel better and requires us to use less energy. We realise you may not always have a reason to smile, but smiling even if you don't feel like it makes you feel happier. Try smiling at yourself in the mirror each morning and you will notice a positive change in your mood. Similarly, laughing makes us feel good too. Try to see the humour in everyday things to help lighten your mood. Read funny books or watch a good comedy to brighten your outlook. This prevents us from taking life too seriously, leaving us feeling positive.

As well as, or instead of, keeping a journal, you may like to fill a book with positive quotes, statements, pictures and humorous, feel-good anecdotes. Look through these every now and then to make you feel better.

Realise that you must believe in yourself. We can't always control things that happen around us, nor can we control other people's actions. Some people are "drains" and are so negative that they drain you just by being in their company. Others are "radiators", in that they radiate positivity and are a pleasure to be around. Now, we can't control everybody, but we can ensure that we radiate positivity and calm. Don't blame others, take responsibility and realise that you are the only person that can give yourself a break. Make your own decisions, be assertive and rise above the need for constant approval of others. Certainly accept their thoughts and feelings, but make allowances for your own ideas, emotions and feelings as well.

Affirmations are a fantastic way to bring about positive change. These are phrases that we repeat on a regular basis. Over time, our mind begins to believe these statements through constant repetition. As simple as it sounds, it really does work. We become what we think and say, so make sure it is positive. Repeat these silently to yourself, say them out loud, even sing them or write them down and pin them up somewhere where you will regularly see them. The key is to practice them regularly throughout the day. Try a classic affirmation such as "day by day, in every way, I am getting better and better". This can be applied to a multitude of situations. Perhaps you would like to replace it with "day by day, in every way, I'm getting stronger and stronger". You could also try a simple phrase such as "I feel good", "I am confident", "I think positive", "all is well" or "I can cope".

Another affirmation that is extremely useful to use during a stressful situation is "relax, take a deep breath, I am in control". You can simply shorten this to "relax", "take a deep breath" or "I am in control", whatever one works best for you. This can be useful just to help us take time to pause and get in control of the situation, enabling us to cope better.

You can also make your own affirmation if none of these are suitable. Always make sure your affirmation is in the present tense. Remember that we want to bring about positive change now, not in the future, so base your affirmation on "I am" not "I will be".

You may like to write your affirmations in your positivity journal, should you decide to keep one. Writing your affirmations helps us to focus on them and memorise them. The more we remind ourselves of them, the more likely we are to believe them and make them part of our mindset. This makes it possible for them to become reality. Write them down as often as you like until you feel you have achieved your goals.

Visualisation can also help promote positive change. We have already learnt how to visualise; try visualising yourself how you want to be and feel. See yourself as already being confident, stronger, full of energy, with less stress, free from pain or whatever you want to achieve. You can visualise this throughout the day or incorporate this into your relaxation visualisation. For example, as you picture yourself lying on the beach, feel your positivity increase as you bask in the sun. If you have any aches or pains, focus on the affected body part, feeling it ease with the warmth of the sun's rays each time you exhale.

By putting our mind in positive mode, we begin to act and look better whilst feeling more upbeat. Positivity creates health and wellbeing, so remember to always stay positive!

One Last Thing

Make time every day to follow the points we have covered. As you see the difference it makes, it will become second nature and part of your daily routine. You will begin to look and feel better, experience less stress as well as more serenity and inner peace. It may seem hard at first. We can hear you screaming "what, no sugar!", "relax – no way, I'm too stressed", "exercise? I'm far too tired", but we assure you that as you start to follow the advice given in this book you will begin to see results. Eating healthy, keeping fit, taking time to relax and looking on the bright side helps accelerate wellbeing and boost energy.

Take your time to introduce these changes to your everyday life. Start by making dietary changes. Try reducing sugar, processed and refined foods whilst eating more fruit and vegetables. Create a good sleep pattern and keep moving through exercise. Learn to consciously and creatively relax. Develop an optimistic, positive attitude. We are sure that as you do this you will see improvements within your body and mind, giving you the incentive to make this your new way of life.

We realise that any change can take time. Work through the suggestions at your own pace. Perhaps you would like to address your diet first, followed by exercise and then introduce relaxation techniques. Alternatively, you may prefer to jump straight in and tackle it all at once. Many people find the thought of adjusting their diet daunting. You may wish initially to ease yourself into change such as cutting down on processed food first, ensuring adequate water intake and eating a healthy breakfast. Perhaps you would then like to introduce healthy snacks, reducing refined foods and then focus on eating healthy evening meals. Making small changes daily soon adds up to big results. Of course, if you prefer, you can tackle it all head on. Do what's best for you, but please keep at it. It takes approximately 21 days for something to become a habit, so let's make it a healthy habit. If you undertake the advice we have provided and carry it out, then it will eventually become your healthy, natural way of life.

The information we have shared with you can greatly boost your health and wellbeing. However, if you have an occasional slip up and eat unhealthily or don't find the time to exercise, don't give yourself a hard time. We are all human and none of us is perfect. Just pick yourself up, dust yourself down and get back on track. Learn from your mistakes so that you know what to do or what not to do next time. Also, remember that if you decide to allow yourself a treat, that's alright too. Enjoy it, don't feel guilty about it, but acknowledge that it should only be an occasional occurrence and shouldn't be a regular part of your diet. Use the tips we have given you on positive thinking to keep up your momentum. Remember that you have all the power you need within you to succeed.

Everybody has the ability to improve themselves. No matter where you are starting from, be it good health or poor health, you can improve your wellbeing by incorporating the information we have provided. We can't work miracles, but we can give you the tools to make the most of yourself. Following the wellbeing advice given allows you to do this. Over time, you will begin to balance body, mind and spirit helping to create health and wellness. You will begin to feel more energised, tranquil and positive. You will cope better with stress and radiate calm.

Remember, you have an amazing ability within yourself to bring about healing in both body and mind. Managing stress, eating well, sleeping better, exercising and thinking positively all combine to create a better, healthier and more relaxed you.

Here's to your health and wellbeing...

Recipes

Taking a wholefood approach to eating is one of the best things you can do for your health. Good food supports the immune system, boosts your health and wellbeing whilst helping you to maintain a healthy weight. However, don't be fooled into thinking wholefoods have to be boring and bland. Just because it's good for you doesn't mean you have to compromise on taste. On the contrary, wholefoods can be both exciting and bursting with flavour.

Here at Holistichem, we believe that food should be enjoyed. We love healthy food, but we also like our food to be interesting and above all taste good. To help you, we've put together some of our favourite and flavoursome recipes. These will give you lots of ideas for healthy meals, snacks, drinks, desserts and cakes (yes, that's right – healthy desserts and cakes!).

Our recipes are quick, simple and easy to make on your own. Try them out; tweak them to suit your tastes and dietary requirements or double the ingredients to make enough to share with family and friends. We give you suggestions for ingredients, but feel free to adapt recipes. For example, you can use dairy-free spread instead of butter and any natural sweetener in place of those we have stated. All our recipes are free from refined sugar. They are also mostly free from gluten, dairy and animal produce. We always provide alternatives if, on occasion, we use any of these ingredients. For example, if we state any foods containing wheat, we also give you gluten-free and/or grain-free options. If we use any animal-based produce, we always list vegetarian/vegan options also. Where possible, we also give egg and nut-free options. We've made sure that our recipes are adaptable, so have fun adjusting them to suit your needs. Where applicable, we've provided both metric and cup measurements for all recipes. For accuracy, we always recommend using metric measurements. A good set of scales is a kitchen essential. However, cup measurements can be quick and handy.

Depending on where you live, this may be the system that you are used to using. Use whichever you feel most comfortable working with. Please note that we use UK ingredient names and some may differ from what you are familiar with if you live elsewhere. For example, courgette is also known as zucchini, coriander as cilantro and self-raising flour as self-rising flour.

We always recommend that, where possible, you try to use organic produce and opt for raw, free-range, sustainably reared and/or grass-fed/pastured varieties. It isn't imperative to use ingredients that are, for example, organic and raw in order to make good dishes, but it does provide you with healthy, pesticide-free food the way nature intended. However, always buy the best from what is available to you and which you can comfortably afford.

You may wish to limit the use of plastic around the house, especially when heating food. Many plastics contain toxins. When heated, these chemicals can actually leach into our food or drinks. Opt for glass or ceramic containers as these are safer. Plastics that are free from BPA are also a good choice.

Remember to take the time to enjoy and savour your food. Never skip or rush your meals. Always eat in an unhurried and relaxing environment. Turn eating into a pleasurable experience. Become conscious of what you are eating. Don't just gulp it down. Enjoy every mouthful. Eat mindfully. Good digestion promotes good health and a wholefood diet gives us the best chance to achieve this.

Go ahead, enjoy experimenting, enjoy cooking, enjoy better health and above all, enjoy your food.

Drinks

Green Juice (serves 1)

This drink is rich in vitamins and minerals and is a highly alkalising vegetable juice, which is great to start the day with or whenever you wish a healthy drink.

1 stalk celery

1 carrot

1 handful lettuce leaves such as Romaine

1 handful spinach, kale or watercress

2"/5cm cucumber

Method: Put ingredients through a juicer and serve.

Tip: If using organic produce, you can simply scrub the vegetables without peeling. If you wish, you can do this for all recipes if using organic fruit and vegetables. You don't need to discard all the leftover pulp. If desired, you can stir some into your juice or add to smoothies, soups and baking to boost the fibre content.

Beetroot and Carrot Juice (serves 1)

Beetroot has fantastic cleansing and purifying properties, helps boost the immune system and fortifies the blood. Abundant in vitamin A and C, iron, potassium and B vitamins, beetroot is also a great energiser. Combined with vitamin A, C, calcium and magnesium-rich carrots, it provides immune-boosting benefits.

2 beetroots

2 carrots

1 stalk celery (optional)

Method: Put ingredients through a juicer and serve.

Carrot and Apple Juice (serves 1)

This juice is a rich source of beta-carotene, vitamin A, quercetin and more. It quenches the thirst at any time of day.

2 carrots

1 apple

1"/2.5cm piece of fresh ginger (optional)

Method: Put ingredients through a juicer and serve.

Tip: Drink fresh juices within 20 minutes to obtain the optimal amount of nutrients. If you want to drink it later, bear in mind that fresh juice oxidises quickly. Store in the fridge in an airtight container. Drink within a few hours and definitely no longer than 24 hours. Ideally, you should drink it immediately as even if properly stored there will be a loss of nutrients. However, this is still better than drinking processed juices. Watch out for oxidisation. Try adding a squeeze of fresh lemon or lime juice to slow down discolouration. If you have a cold press/masticating juicer, you can store your juice in the fridge for up to 48 hours. This type of juicer, also known as a slow juicer, preserves the nutritional content for longer than juices made with a centrifugal juicer.

Nut Milk (makes approximately 3 cups)

Dairy-free nut milk is a great alternative to cows' milk and, whilst available to buy, it is also very easy to make at home. Use as a non-dairy milk replacement in smoothies, warm drinks and baking. Tastes great mixed with freshly squeezed juices as well as with healthy wholegrain/gluten-free cereals and porridge. Use organic and/or raw nuts, if possible, but any unsalted varieties are acceptable. You can also make this using seeds such as sesame, pumpkin and hemp seeds.

150g/1 cup nuts such as almonds, cashews or hazelnuts
720ml/3 cups filtered or mineral water
2 dates (optional)
¼ teaspoon ground cinnamon or vanilla essence/powder (optional)
Pinch of sea salt (optional)

Method: Cover nuts with some water and leave to soak overnight to soften. After soaking, rinse nuts and blend along with the filtered water. Add in optional ingredients, if using. Process until fully blended. Pour nut milk through a sieve, muslin cloth or nut milk bag to separate the pulp from the liquid. Once strained, store in an airtight container in the fridge. Keeps for 3-5 days.

Tip: Soak nuts for at least 8-12 hours. Soaking helps to remove the naturally occurring phytic acid and also softens the nuts. This allows for them to be more easily blended. You can use the nut pulp to add to smoothies and baking to provide a healthy boost of protein. If you don't mind the texture, you can leave the pulp in the milk for added fibre. You can also sweeten this milk with any liquid-based natural sweetener such as agave nectar or a few drops of liquid stevia.

Berry Smoothie (serves 1)

A smoothie makes an ideal quick breakfast and is great to keep you going between meals. This smoothie is packed full of vitamins B, C, E, fibre, protein and slow releasing carbohydrates.

1 handful berries such as raspberries or blueberries
4 tablespoons unsweetened natural yoghurt or coconut yoghurt
240ml/1 cup almond, coconut, oat or rice milk
1 teaspoon barley grass or wheatgrass (optional)
1 tablespoon of gluten-free oats (optional)
1 tablespoon hemp powder (optional)
1 teaspoon seeds such as pumpkin, ground flax or chia (optional)
Method: Add ingredients to blender and process until smooth and drink immediately. If you plan to drink it later, transfer to an airtight container and keep cool, preferably refrigerated. Smoothies are best consumed within 24 hours.
Tip: You can use either fresh or frozen berries when making smoothies. This helps to keep them chilled and will give a thicker consistency. Try replacing some, or all, of the milk with some freshly squeezed juice such as apple, carrot or a combination of both. You can add any superfood powder instead of those suggested. You can do this for any of the smoothie recipes.

Green Smoothie (serves 1)

Refreshing and tasty, this nutrient packed salad-in-a-glass smoothie is ideal in the morning or throughout the day.

1 banana
1 handful of green grapes (optional)
1 handful spinach leaves, kale or lettuce
1 stalk celery
240ml/1 cup filtered or mineral water

Method: Add ingredients to blender and process with water until smooth. Depending on the speed of your blender, you may have to chop tougher vegetables, such as celery, before adding to help it break them down. You may have to add more water to help loosen the mixture and to reach your desired consistency. Drink immediately.

Tip: It's a good idea to vary your leafy green vegetables. Whilst very good for you, spinach also contains naturally occurring oxalic acid, which can affect the absorption of vitamins and minerals. It's best to rotate your greens to ensure variety and maximum nutrient uptake. You may find that the leafy greens create a strong taste. As you begin to drink your green smoothie on a regular basis, your taste buds will adjust and you will come to enjoy the clean, green flavour. You can also use other liquids in green smoothies such as coconut water, non-dairy milk and green tea.

Chocolate Banana Smoothie (serves 1)

This delicious smoothie is rich in minerals, such as magnesium and calcium, thanks to the banana and tahini. Enjoy at any time, but it is especially good as an afternoon energy boost. So much healthier than reaching for a biscuit and much more enjoyable too. Tastes just like chocolate milk, the only difference being that this is good for you.

1 banana

1 tablespoon tahini

1 tablespoon raw cacao powder or carob powder

240ml/1 cup almond, coconut, oat or rice milk

120ml/½ cup milk kefir (optional; if using, reduce milk quantity to 120ml/½ cup)

Method: Whizz ingredients together in blender until smooth and serve.

Tip: Raw cacao powder is rich in nutrients. If you don't have this, then you can substitute it with unsweetened cocoa powder.

Banana and Coconut Smoothie (serves 1)

Packed full of potassium, calcium, vitamins and antioxidants, this smoothie is satisfying at any time of day. It is free from dairy, which makes it ideal for those with an allergy to cows' milk as well as vegans. Of course, it's suitable for everyone else too.

1 banana

1 handful berries such as raspberries or blueberries

1 tablespoon raw coconut oil

240ml/1 cup coconut milk or coconut water

1 tablespoon seeds such as ground flax or chia (optional)

Method: Blend ingredients together and serve.

Tip: You can also use frozen bananas. To freeze bananas, simply peel, cut into chunks and freeze in an airtight container. This allows you to always keep a supply of ripe bananas. Frozen fruits also help to thicken smoothies. This smoothie also makes a great pudding/smoothie bowl. Simply reduce or omit the liquids and blend to make a thick pudding-style consistency that can be eaten at breakfast, after dinner or as a snack. You can add a variety of toppings such as nuts, seeds and fruit.

Breakfasts

Muesli (serves 1)

This muesli-style breakfast is a delicious way to get protein, slow release carbohydrates and a fruit portion in one go. It also provides a satisfying start to the morning.

1 tablespoon gluten-free oats

1 apple, grated

1 tablespoon flaked almonds and/or seeds such as pumpkin or sunflower

Sprinkling of ground cinnamon (optional)

Method: Combine ingredients and serve with milk of your choice.

Tip: You can easily increase the quantity of the dry ingredients to make a supply, saving preparation time in the morning. Store in an airtight container and simply add fruit and milk to the mixture before serving.

Quinoa Porridge (serves 1)

A warming bowl of quinoa porridge sets you up for the day, providing fibre, protein, vitamins and minerals. It is low-glycaemic; therefore, will not spike sugar levels. It makes for a healthier alternative to many conventional sugar-laden cereals. This dish is easy on the digestive system and is also free from gluten and dairy.

40g/½ cup quinoa flakes

240ml/1 cup filtered or mineral water and/or almond or rice milk

Pinch of sea salt

1 teaspoon raw honey or agave nectar, berries, nuts, seeds, ground cinnamon or chopped dates (optional)

Method: Add quinoa flakes and liquid to pan. Bring quinoa flakes and liquid to the boil, reduce heat and stir constantly until desired consistency. Top with a choice of fruit, spice, nuts, seeds, natural sweetener or simply serve on its own.

Overnight Oats (serves 1)

Oats provide slow releasing carbohydrates and lots of heart-friendly nutrients. They are a good source of soluble fibre that is easily digested. Adding fruit provides antioxidants, vitamins and minerals, whilst nuts and seeds gives a protein hit. This breakfast dish is quick and easy and as it is prepared the night before, there is no excuse for not having a healthy and filling start to the day.

40g/½ cup gluten-free oats

120ml/½ cup almond, coconut, oat or rice milk

120ml/½ cup unsweetened natural yoghurt or coconut yoghurt

Raw cacao powder, nut butter, banana, apple, berries, nuts, seeds, agave nectar or coconut nectar (optional)

Method: Combine ingredients. If using raw cacao powder and/or nut butter, add now. Place in fridge overnight to allow liquids to absorb. Top with choice of fruit, nuts, seeds and/or natural sweetener. Toppings can be added at night, when making, or in the morning upon serving.

Chia Seed Pudding (serves 1)

Chia seeds are a wonderful source of fibre, minerals and essential fatty acids. Along with goji berries, this pudding provides antioxidants and helps keep you full for longer. Ideal for breakfast or any time of the day. For a healthy chocolate treat, add some raw cacao or carob powder and natural sweetener.

4 tablespoons chia seeds

180ml/¾ cup coconut milk

1 teaspoon coconut sugar or agave nectar

1 handful dried goji berries (optional)

1 teaspoon raw cacao powder or carob powder (optional)

Method: Add coconut milk to seeds and stir until mixture thickens. Add in natural sweetener. If using berries and/or cacao/carob powder, add these also. Allow to sit for 10 minutes or overnight in fridge.

Tip: You can also use filtered/mineral water instead of the coconut milk. It won't be as creamy but still tastes nice.

Mini Frittata Muffin (serves 1)

This mini frittata provides a healthy hit of protein to start the morning off right and is extremely quick to prepare. It can be made in advance and stored in the fridge for the next day. Ideal for snacking on, it is also good to have on hand throughout the day. You can easily make a bigger batch by multiplying the ingredients.

1 free-range egg (preferably organic)

Selection of vegetables such as onions or peppers, chopped

Sea salt and freshly ground black pepper, to taste

Method: Preheat oven to 180°C/350°F/Gas Mark 4. Beat the egg in a bowl and set aside. Add a small amount of chopped vegetables to one muffin cup. Pour beaten egg over vegetables and season with salt and pepper. Bake in oven for 15 minutes or until egg is thoroughly cooked and golden on top. Can be eaten hot or cold.

Tip: For an egg-free option, try substituting the egg with silken tofu or vegan egg replacer.

Soups

Detox Soup (serves 4)

This alkalising soup is packed full of antioxidants and is perfect for helping you offload toxins and lighten up. Tastes great at any time of the year, it is light and delicate during the summer yet warming enough for winter. It is also ideal for soothing delicate digestive systems as it helps to cleanse and balance from within.

1 leek, chopped

1 bag (approximately 120g/3 cups) watercress, spinach and rocket

1 potato, chopped

600ml/2½ cups vegetable stock

1 tablespoon miso paste (optional)

Sea salt and freshly ground black pepper, to taste

Method: Sauté leek for a few minutes until soft. Add leafy green vegetables, potato and vegetable stock. If using miso, add this now. Bring to the boil and simmer for about 20-30 minutes until potato is cooked. Blend for a smoother consistency. Season and serve.

Tip: You can use any leafy green vegetable in this soup. Kale and spring greens also taste good. Whilst leafy green vegetables are good for you, it is a good idea to rotate them to ensure variety and maximum nutrient absorption.

Sweet Potato Soup (serves 4)

Bursting with vitamin C and fibre, this filling soup is ideal for lunch or as part of your evening meal. It is also rich in vitamin E, beta-carotene and B vitamins.

1 leek, chopped
2 sweet potatoes, chopped
1 potato, chopped (optional)
600ml/2½ cups vegetable stock
Sea salt and freshly ground black pepper, to taste
Swirl of unsweetened Greek yoghurt or coconut cream (optional)
Method: Sauté leek until soft. Add potatoes and stock. Bring to the boil and simmer until potatoes are soft, approximately 25 minutes. Blend or mash until desired consistency. Season and serve. Add a swirl of yoghurt/coconut cream to each bowl, if desired.
Tip: Add a pinch of good quality salt to leeks when sautéing to help release natural juices. This also works well with onions. Try roasting potatoes in a little extra virgin olive oil before adding to pot for a richer, fuller flavour.

Pea Soup (serves 4)

A good source of vegetable protein and fibre, this pea soup is quick and easy to make. It is rich in antioxidants, vitamins and minerals such as vitamin C, folic acid and B vitamins.

1 leek, chopped

400g/scant 2 cups frozen peas

1 parsnip, chopped (optional)

600ml/2½ cups vegetable stock

Sea salt and freshly ground black pepper, to taste

½ teaspoon ground coriander (optional)

Method: Sauté leek until soft. Add peas. Add parsnip, if using. This will make a thicker soup. Add stock, bring to the boil and simmer until vegetables are cooked, approximately 10 minutes/25 minutes, if using parsnip. Add coriander, if using, and cook for a further few minutes. Blend until smooth. Season and serve.

Lentil Soup (serves 4)

Rich in B vitamins, carbohydrates and proteins, this hearty lentil soup will keep you warm on the coldest of days. It is very filling, making it a satisfying meal served with wholegrain/gluten-free bread and/or salad.

1 leek, chopped

1 stalk celery, chopped

1 carrot, chopped

225g/1 cup red lentils

600ml/2½ cups vegetable or chicken stock

Sea salt and freshly ground black pepper, to taste

Method: Sauté leek and celery until soft. Add carrot. Rinse lentils thoroughly and add to pot. Add stock and bring to the boil. Simmer until lentils and vegetables are soft, approximately 30-40 minutes. Add more stock if needed as lentils absorb liquid quickly. Blend until desired consistency. Season and serve.

Tip: You can soak the lentils for easier digestion. Simply soak in water overnight, rinse and cook in fresh water. This technique can be used for all recipes containing pulses and/or grains. If you are a meat-eater, using leftover chicken bones from a roast makes a good base for a homemade stock. Bones that have been roasted add a richer, more palatable flavour to the stock. You can also use any type of bone or cuts of meat on the bone. Ham, beef and lamb all taste good. Just make sure you use those from good quality, preferably organic and/or grass-fed/pastured sources. You can substitute any of the stock used in the soup recipes to suit your own taste and requirements.

Butternut Squash and Butter Bean Soup (serves 4)

Butternut squash is bursting with antioxidants, vitamin A and B vitamins. Butter beans are rich in both carbohydrates and protein, providing vitamin A, iron, calcium and zinc. This is a lovely warming soup.

1 leek, chopped

1 butternut squash, chopped

2 carrots, chopped

600ml/2½ cups vegetable stock

400g/14oz can butter beans (alternatively, use 1½ cups cooked butter beans)

Method: Sauté leek until soft. Add butternut squash and carrot to the pot. Add stock and bring to the boil. Simmer until vegetables are soft, approximately 20-25 minutes. Then add butter beans and allow to heat through. Blend or mash until desired consistency. Season and serve.

Tip: This also tastes great using roasted butternut squash. Simply roast the squash and follow the recipe above, adding this in towards the end of cooking. If beans are not well tolerated, you can omit them. The soup still tastes nice without them.

Main Meals

Courgette and Lemon Pasta (serves 2)

Courgettes are rich in vitamin C and contain manganese, which is good for helping to regulate blood sugar levels. Lemons are wonderfully alkalising and a good source of vitamin C. Enjoy this served over wholewheat, rice, corn or spelt pasta.

150-200g/¾-1 cup cooked pasta

1 courgette, grated

Juice and zest of ½ unwaxed lemon

Drizzle of extra virgin olive oil

Sea salt and freshly ground black pepper, to taste

Method: Add courgette to cooked pasta with lemon juice, zest, olive oil and season to taste. Can be served warm in which case the heat from the pasta will gently warm the courgette. Alternatively, this can also be eaten once pasta has cooled.

Tomato Pasta Sauce (serves 2)

A good source of lycopene, beta-carotene and vitamin C and E, this sauce is great served with wholewheat, rice, corn or spelt pasta. It also makes a good Bolognese sauce and freezes well.

1 onion, chopped

1 clove garlic, crushed or ⅛ teaspoon garlic powder

½ teaspoon dried basil

½ teaspoon dried oregano

400g/14oz can chopped tomatoes

1 teaspoon tomato purée

Vegetable stock, to taste (optional)

Drizzle of agave nectar (optional)

Method: Sauté onion until soft. Add garlic, herbs, chopped tomatoes and tomato purée. Bring to the boil and simmer until liquid thickens and reduces, approximately 25 minutes. If a thinner sauce is preferred, add a little vegetable stock until desired consistency. A drizzle of agave nectar can be added for a sweeter sauce. Pour over cooked pasta.

Tip: If garlic causes digestive symptoms, you can replace it with a garlic-infused oil. Opt for a good quality, cold pressed oil and, where possible, organic. You can also sauté a peeled clove of garlic in some oil for approximately 5 minutes. Stir frequently and then discard the garlic. This provides flavour without unpleasant side effects. Alternatively, you can use black garlic. This is kinder on the digestive system and often better tolerated. You can do any of these for all recipes that include garlic.

Creamy Basil Pasta Sauce (serves 2)

Basil has antioxidant, anti-inflammatory and anti-bacterial properties. It also helps to aid digestion and is a rich source of lutein and zeaxanthin, which is good for eye health. Cashew nuts contain protein, monounsaturated fats, magnesium, zinc and B vitamins. Use unsalted cashew nuts and, if possible, opt for organic and/or raw varieties. This sauce has a lovely creamy texture making it ideal served over wholewheat/ gluten-free pasta.

75g/½ cup cashew nuts

400ml/14oz can coconut milk

1 tablespoon butter (preferably organic and/or grass-fed) or dairy-free spread

2 cloves garlic, crushed or ¼ teaspoon garlic powder

1½ teaspoons sea salt

1 large handful fresh basil

Method: Cover cashew nuts with water and soak overnight to soften. Once softened, place in a blender. Blend cashew nuts with coconut milk, butter/dairy-free spread, garlic and salt until thick and smooth. Add in the basil leaves and blend until finely chopped and mixed together. Pour the sauce over cooked pasta. Stir to mix.

Tip: If you have a high-speed blender, you can add the cashews to the blender without soaking. However, soaking them will help to reduce the phytic acid and make them more digestible.

Nutty Noodles with Mixed Vegetables (serves 2-3)

This tasty noodle dish is the perfect balance of healthy carbohydrates, protein and fats, thanks to the noodles and nut butter. Be sure to use wholegrain varieties or gluten-free noodles for the healthiest form of carbohydrates. You can also make this with spiralized vegetable noodles, if preferred. This is very quick to prepare and creates a delicious, nutrient-rich dish in a flash.

2-4 tablespoons cashew or almond butter

60ml/¼ cup toasted sesame oil

60ml/¼ cup Sweet Freedom, agave nectar or raw honey

1 tablespoon raw apple cider vinegar

1 teaspoon tamari or Bragg Liquid Aminos

300g/3 cups wholewheat or rice noodles

Selection of vegetables such as onions, peppers or courgettes, chopped

Sea salt and freshly ground black pepper, to taste

Method: In a bowl, combine nut butter, toasted sesame oil, natural sweetener, apple cider vinegar and tamari/liquid aminos and stir until smooth. In a separate pan, cook selected vegetables in oil until softened. To this, add cooked noodles and heat together. Pour over sauce, stir, heat through and then serve. Alternatively, refrigerate and serve chilled.

Tip: For a nut-free version, try using tahini or a seed butter such as pumpkin or sunflower.

Chicken and Tomatoes (serves 2)

Chicken provides low-fat protein along with vitamin C and lycopene from the tomatoes. It is also a good source of tryptophan, which helps to elevate mood and promote better sleep. Serve this with brown rice for a filling meal. You can always make this with a meat alternative such as tofu or Quorn.

2 chicken breasts (preferably free-range, organic and/or pastured)
2 handfuls plum tomatoes
1 clove garlic, crushed or ⅛ teaspoon garlic powder
1 handful fresh basil
Sea salt and freshly ground black pepper, to taste
Drizzle of extra virgin olive oil
Method: Wash and halve tomatoes and add to baking tray. Wash and chop basil. Add this along with garlic. Place chicken on top of tomato layer and season. Drizzle with olive oil and bake at 180°C/350°F/Gas mark 4 for 30-40 minutes or until chicken is thoroughly cooked.

Salmon and Rice Salad (serves 2)

Salmon is a fantastic source of omega-3 fatty acids and brown rice provides B vitamins. Salmon also contains valuable levels of the antioxidant selenium. This can be served cold and is ideal to prepare for lunch the night before, especially if you have some leftover salmon from your evening meal. If serving cold, resistant starch is formed as the cooked rice cools. This provides prebiotics and helps to lower blood sugar levels. This dish can also be made without fish if you prefer a vegetarian/vegan option. Substituting the rice for quinoa works well too.

200g/1 cup cooked brown rice
2 fillets cooked salmon, flaked (preferably organic/wild and sustainably reared)
1 handful sugar snap peas
Dash of tamari or Bragg Liquid Aminos
½ teaspoon Chinese 5 Spice (optional)
1 handful edamame beans (optional)
Drizzle of extra virgin olive oil

Method: Flake the fish. Combine with brown rice and chopped raw sugar snap peas. Add tamari/liquid aminos, spice and beans, if using, and drizzle over olive oil. Mix together and serve immediately. If serving cold, allow to cool and store in fridge until ready to serve.

Tip: This also tastes great served with cauliflower rice for a grain-free option. Simply, chop cauliflower florets in a food processor, lightly sauté in a pan to heat through. Serve immediately or allow to cool. Alternatively, cauliflower rice can also be eaten raw.

Coconut Curry Sauce (serves 3-4)

This creamy sauce is a dairy-free alternative to commercial curry sauces. Coconut milk is rich in minerals such as phosphorus and magnesium. This is ideal served with vegetables, tofu, Quorn, fish, chicken or lean beef. Serve with brown rice, cauliflower rice, millet or rice noodles.

1 tablespoon rapeseed oil

Dash of tamari or coconut aminos

Pinch of chilli flakes

1 teaspoon mild curry powder

1 teaspoon ground turmeric

1 teaspoon coconut sugar or xylitol (preferably non-GMO and sustainably sourced)

1 teaspoon sea salt

400ml/14oz can coconut milk

Method: Heat oil and add tamari/coconut aminos. Add spices, natural sweetener and salt, then mix to a paste. Sauté for a few minutes, then add coconut milk. Heat gently. You can then add vegetables, meat, fish or meat substitute of your choice and simmer until cooked. Alternatively, use as a pour over sauce.

Raw Spinach Pesto (serves 2-3)

Spinach is a wonderful source of iron, B vitamins and folic acid. Making this sauce with raw spinach preserves the nutrients that would otherwise be destroyed during cooking. Serve with wholewheat, rice, buckwheat or spelt pasta. You may also like to serve it with raw or lightly cooked spiralized vegetable noodles.

2 large handfuls spinach

1 handful pine nuts or walnuts

1 clove garlic, crushed or ⅛ teaspoon garlic powder

Drizzle of extra virgin olive oil

2"/5cm Pecorino Romano or dairy-free alternative, grated

Sea salt and freshly ground black pepper, to taste

Method: Add all the ingredients to a food processor or blender. Process until smooth and ingredients combined. Keep adding a drizzle of olive oil until desired consistency. Season and serve over warm pasta. Heat from the pasta will gently warm the sauce. Alternatively, serve cold.

Tip: Try using different leaves such as basil and rocket. You can also use different nuts and seeds such as cashews or sunflower seeds. Where possible, opt for organic and/or raw varieties.

Lentil Bolognese (serves 3-4)

Lentils are a fantastic source of B vitamins, protein and fibre. They also help to regulate blood sugar and are very low in fat. Serving this with brown rice, spelt spaghetti, spiralized vegetables or as part of a wholegrain/gluten-free lasagne provides a complete vegetable protein. This is suitable for freezing.

115g/⅔ cup red lentils

1 onion, diced

2 peppers, 1 chopped/1 puréed

1 carrot, grated

400g/14oz can chopped tomatoes

300ml/1¼ cups vegetable stock

2 cloves garlic, crushed or ¼ teaspoon garlic powder

1 teaspoon dried basil

1 teaspoon dried oregano

Method: Rinse lentils thoroughly. Sauté the onion and chopped pepper until softened. Add the lentils, carrot, tomatoes, puréed pepper, stock, garlic, basil and oregano to pot. Bring to the boil and simmer covered for 30 minutes or until the lentils are soft but not mushy. You may require to add more stock as lentils absorb liquid quickly.

Tip: This also tastes great made into a vegetarian Shepherd's Pie. Use the lentil Bolognese as the base and top with mashed potato/sweet potato. Simply bake until the potato is browned and the dish is cooked through. You can also top with mashed cauliflower for a low-starch option.

Chickpea Curry (serves 3-4)

Chickpeas are a good source of vegetable protein and are rich in antioxidants. Packed full of fibre, chickpeas are beneficial to digestion, thanks to their substantial levels of insoluble fibre. This is a tasty dish that is great served with brown rice, cauliflower rice or quinoa.

1 onion, chopped

1 pepper, chopped

400g/14oz can chickpeas (alternatively, use 2 cups cooked chickpeas)

50g/scant ½ cup frozen peas

150g/5oz can sweetcorn (preferably non-GMO)

400g/14oz can chopped tomatoes

400ml/14oz can coconut milk

1 clove garlic, crushed or ⅛ teaspoon garlic powder

1 teaspoon fresh ginger, grated

1 teaspoon ground coriander

1 teaspoon ground cumin

Method: Sauté the onion and pepper until softened. Add the rest of ingredients. Bring to the boil and simmer for 15 minutes. Serve with wholegrain of choice.

Quinoa (serves 3-4)

Although quinoa may look like a grain, it is actually a seed and is naturally free from gluten. It is also a complete vegetable protein and is rich in B vitamins and minerals such as phosphorous, potassium, zinc and selenium. This makes an ideal lunch or main meal. Can be served alone or along with chicken, tuna, tofu or salad.

150g/⅔ cup uncooked quinoa
300ml/1¼ cups filtered or mineral water
1 vegetable stock cube or 1 teaspoon vegetable bouillon (optional)
1 onion, chopped
1 pepper, chopped
1 courgette, chopped
Drizzle of extra virgin olive oil
1 teaspoon dried parsley
1 teaspoon dried rosemary
1 teaspoon dried basil

Method: Rinse quinoa thoroughly. Place in a pan of water and bring to the boil. Alternatively, you may wish to add a stock cube/bouillon to add more flavour. You may need to add more liquid if absorbed during cooking. Sauté the onion, pepper and courgette until softened. Drizzle olive oil over the quinoa and add the parsley, rosemary and basil, mixing well. Add the pepper, onion and courgette to the quinoa. Can be served warm or cold, after chilling in the fridge.

Tip: You can also cook quinoa in bone broth such as homemade chicken stock. You can do this with any grains or pulses as bone broth helps to make them more digestible.

Gravy (serves 3-4)

This gravy is a perfect accompaniment to a variety of wholefood dishes. Unlike conventional gravies, this is free from gluten and yeast. It is great served with vegetarian dishes, such as our vegetable casserole, as well as over good quality meat. You can also make this with any unrefined flour such as spelt flour.

2 tablespoons of oil such as rapeseed or extra virgin olive oil
1 onion, chopped
2 tablespoons gluten-free flour
1 clove garlic, crushed or ⅛ teaspoon garlic powder
480ml/2 cups vegetable stock
2 tablespoons tamari or Bragg Liquid Aminos

Method: Sauté the onion in the oil for 5 minutes. Add the flour and cook for a further 5-10 minutes until the onion is soft and browned. Add the garlic and gradually stir in the vegetable stock. Bring to the boil and simmer for about 10 minutes. Add the tamari/liquid aminos and stir well. Strain, if you like, or serve as is.

Vegetable Casserole (serves 3-4)

This hearty casserole is packed full of nutrient-rich vegetables. Onions are rich in vitamin C and quercetin. Choose from a variety of root vegetables to add to this warming and nourishing dish. Wonderfully filling, this is ideal comfort food without the usual stodge. As with most of our main meals, any leftovers makes for a satisfying lunch the next day.

1 onion, chopped

Selection of vegetables such as carrots, potatoes, parsnips or sweet potatoes, chopped

600ml/2½ cups vegetable stock

Method: Sauté the onion until softened. Add the rest of selected vegetables and stock. If required, you can adjust the quantity of stock to suit the amount of vegetables used. Bring to the boil and simmer for approximately 20 minutes or until softened. Once vegetables are tender, drain stock. Reserve stock to use as a basis for vegetarian gravy as per previous recipe. Once gravy is made, pour back over vegetables and serve.

Tip: On occasion, meat eaters can also add sausages along with vegetables. Choose good quality pork, preferably organic and/or pastured and sustainably reared. Look for sausages that are free from gluten and made with no added water to ensure you are eating the best quality available. Try adding a meat substitute, such as tofu or Quorn, if you prefer a meat-free option.

Vegetarian Chilli (serves 3-4)

Bulgur wheat is a natural wholegrain and is high in fibre and healthy carbohydrates. It contains minerals such as manganese, phosphorous and iron. It is also a rich source of B vitamins. Tomatoes provide antioxidants and lycopene, whilst kidney beans are a good source of vegetable protein. For a gluten-free option, you can easily substitute bulgur wheat for quinoa. Ideal as a main meal, this is also great to take for lunch the next day.

120ml/½ cup passata

95g/½ cup uncooked bulgur wheat

1 onion, chopped

2 peppers, chopped

150g/5oz can sweetcorn (preferably non-GMO)

2 x 400g/14oz cans chopped tomatoes

400g/14oz can kidney beans (alternatively, use 2 cups cooked kidney beans)

2 cloves garlic, crushed or ¼ teaspoon garlic powder

2 teaspoons chilli powder

½ teaspoon ground cumin

½ teaspoon dried oregano

Method: In a saucepan, heat the passata and bring to the boil. Remove from heat and stir in the bulgur wheat. Cover and let stand for about 30 minutes or until the passata is absorbed. Meanwhile, in another pot, mix the remaining ingredients. Cook over a medium heat, stirring frequently, until vegetables are tender. Stir in bulgur wheat and heat through.

Tip: Try replacing kidney beans with another type of bean such as borlotti beans.

Houmous Tofu (serves 2)

Tofu provides a good source of vegetable protein and phytoestrogens. These are also present in houmous due to its chickpea content. Chickpeas also contain fibre, folate, magnesium and potassium. Tofu is also great for lowering cholesterol levels. Serve with brown rice and vegetables. For a grain-free option, serve with cauliflower rice.

1 pack extra firm tofu (preferably organic and non-GMO)
2 tablespoons tamari or Bragg Liquid Aminos
1 tablespoon agave nectar or coconut nectar
1 tablespoon raw apple cider vinegar
120ml/½ cup filtered or mineral water
2 teaspoons dried rosemary
1 teaspoon dried thyme
1 teaspoon dried parsley
3 tablespoons houmous

Method: Drain the tofu and press to remove any excess liquid. Once drained, chop into 1" cubes. Meanwhile, in a separate dish, mix the rest of the ingredients to create the marinade. Place the tofu in the marinade; then gently stir until all is thoroughly covered. Cover and let sit for at least 30 minutes. For the best flavour, leave the tofu in the marinade overnight. Once marinated, spoon the houmous over the tofu and cover thoroughly. Aim for a thick coating over each piece of tofu. Bake in a preheated oven at 350°F/180°C/Gas mark 4 for 30 minutes.

Sweets

Cinnamon Cookies (makes 16)

These cookies are a delicious, healthy treat and are a winner with everybody. Made with spelt flour, these melt-in-the-mouth cookies are kind on the digestive tract. Spelt is an ideal alternative to refined wheat. It is low-gluten and rich in fibre, vitamins and minerals, including B vitamins, magnesium, copper and iron.

225g/1 cup wholegrain spelt flour
½ teaspoon gluten-free baking powder
2 teaspoons ground cinnamon
75ml/⅓ cup raw honey or agave nectar
120ml/½ cup unrefined sunflower oil

Method: Preheat oven to 190°C/375°F/Gas mark 5. Mix all the ingredients, dry first and then liquid. Place spoonfuls on an oiled tray or silicone tray. Bake in oven for 8 to 12 minutes. Allow to cool on a wire rack.

Tip: For an entirely gluten-free version, you can replace the spelt flour with a gluten-free variety of flour.

Pancakes (makes 5 large or 10 small)

Pancakes are usually made with refined wheat, cows' milk and sugar. These pancakes are a healthier, tasty alternative that are free from gluten, dairy and refined sugar. Enjoy these for a weekend breakfast or as a simple snack between meals. Serve warm, drizzled with natural maple syrup, agave/coconut nectar, berries or 100% fruit spread.

240g/1 cup gluten-free self-raising flour
30g/¼ cup coconut sugar or xylitol (preferably non-GMO and sustainably sourced)
240ml/1 cup almond, coconut, oat or rice milk
1 free-range egg (preferably organic)

Method: Add ingredients, dry first and then liquid. Mix until batter is smooth. In an oiled pan, add mixture to form pancake shapes. Cook either side until golden brown and fluffy in the middle. This will only take a few minutes per side.

Tip: For egg-free pancakes, swap the egg for a vegan egg replacer. For a grain-free version, you can substitute the flour for 30g/¼ cup coconut flour whilst increasing to four eggs and omitting the milk. Depending on the size of each pancake, the grain-free version may yield a slightly smaller batch.

Mug Cake (serves 1)

This simple grain-free, protein-rich cake is easy to make and is perfect when you want to whip up a quick, healthy treat. We don't recommend using your microwave all the time for health reasons, but this is one occasion where it is acceptable and is ideal for when nothing but cake will do.

3 tablespoons ground almonds

1 tablespoon coconut sugar or unsweetened desiccated coconut

1 tablespoon raw cacao powder

1 tablespoon almond, coconut, oat or rice milk

1 free-range egg (preferably organic)

Method: In a cup, mix together ingredients, dry first and then liquid. Microwave for 1½ minutes on high power.

Tip: For an egg-free option, substitute with a chia or flax egg replacer.

Oat and Nut Butter Squares (makes approximately 12)

These no-bake squares are quick and very easy to make. The oats provide a sustained release of healthy carbohydrates, while the nut butter supplies nutrient-dense protein and fats. These are great as a nutritious treat and are ideal as a snack between meals.

240g/3 cups gluten-free oats

240g/1 cup nut butter such as cashew or almond butter

120ml/½ cup brown rice syrup, raw honey or agave nectar

1 handful seeds such as sunflower, pumpkin or chia (optional)

Method: Melt the nut butter and natural sweetener in a pan over a low heat. Remove from heat once melted and add in the oats. Add seeds, if using. Mix until ingredients are combined. Pour onto a baking tray lined with greaseproof paper. Spread evenly until around 1" in thickness. Store in the fridge to harden. This should take between 30 minutes to 1 hour depending on the temperature of your fridge. Once cooled and hardened, cut into squares. Store in an airtight container in the fridge.

Tip: Try substituting the nut butter for any seed butter to make a nut-free version.

Carob Crispies (makes approximately 10)

These lovely little cakes are an enjoyable treat and also make a nice, healthy homemade gift. Popular with all ages, these go down well at parties for kids and grown-ups alike. Carob powder is an excellent chocolate alternative. It is free from caffeine and contains antioxidants, calcium and iron.

90g/3 cups unsweetened puffed rice or unsweetened wholegrain cereal

3 tablespoons raw coconut oil

2 tablespoons raw honey or Sweet Freedom

65g/⅓ cup carob powder

Method: Melt coconut oil and natural sweetener in saucepan. Add carob powder and mix well until dissolved. Add puffed rice or wholegrain cereal and mix well. Place spoonfuls in greaseproof paper cases. Refrigerate for 1 hour.

Tip: If desired, raw cacao powder can be used instead of carob powder. You can replace the honey/Sweet Freedom with any natural sweetener. Use a liquid-based sweetener to help the mixture stick together.

Raw Chocolate Truffles (makes approximately 20 balls)

These decadent little truffles are a healthier alternative to sugary sweets. The honey/brown rice syrup gives them a natural sweetness, whilst the coconut oil and nuts provide healthy fats and protein. Use unsalted cashew nuts and, where possible, opt for organic and/or raw varieties. Enjoy these as an occasional treat or make them as an edible gift to give.

250g/scant 2 cups cashew nuts
3 tablespoons raw cacao powder
Pinch of sea salt
3 tablespoons raw coconut oil
4 tablespoons raw honey or brown rice syrup

Method: Grind nuts, cacao powder and salt together until fine. Add coconut oil and natural sweetener. Mix well to form dough; if a little dry, add an extra tablespoon coconut oil. Roll into balls and store in the fridge. Serve once firm.

Tip: Try using different nuts; almonds work well. Also, try replacing the honey/brown rice syrup with agave/coconut nectar. If you wish, you can add a superfood powder to the truffles. Simply add in a teaspoon of powder, such as baobab, barley grass or hemp, to the mixture before shaping into balls.

Avocado Delight (serves 1)

Avocados are a fantastic source of vitamin E and essential fatty acids, which are great for the immune system, heart and skin. This is a quick, healthy sweet treat.

1 avocado

2 teaspoons raw cacao powder or carob powder

60ml/¼ cup coconut milk

1 teaspoon coconut sugar or xylitol (preferably non-GMO and sustainably sourced)

Method: Halve and peel avocado and add to blender with cacao/carob powder, coconut milk and natural sweetener. Blend until smooth and creamy. Serve immediately.

Tip: For a butterscotch flavour, try using lucuma powder instead of cacao/carob powder. Raw honey or agave nectar also works well. Simply use a drizzle to replace the coconut sugar/xylitol.

Halva-Style Tahini (serves 1)

Tahini is simply creamed sesame seeds and is rich in minerals and protein. This is ideal when only something sweet will suffice. Serve alone or eat with raw vegetable cruditiés. Tastes good spread on wholegrain/gluten-free bread, crackers and oatcakes too.

4 tablespoons tahini

½ teaspoon raw honey

1 teaspoon raw cacao powder or carob powder (optional)

Method: Mix tahini and honey together until combined. Add cacao/carob powder, if using. Serve immediately.

Tip: For a firmer texture, refrigerate for 1 hour before serving. Quantities can be increased if you wish to make a large batch.

Banana Choc-Nut Ice Cream (serves 2)

This delicious frozen dessert is a great source of protein, vitamins and minerals as well as natural sweetness. Conventional ice cream is made primarily of fat and sugar, not to mention lots of unnatural ingredients. This ice cream treat is lovely and even provides a fruit portion.

2 bananas

2 tablespoons almond butter

2 tablespoons raw cacao powder

Method: Blend all ingredients in a food processor or blender until smooth consistency. Pour into an airtight container and freeze. After 1-2 hours, take out of the freezer, stir to stop ice crystals forming and then freeze until needed.

Tip: To serve instantly, try making this with frozen bananas. Simply blend frozen banana chunks with other ingredients and serve immediately.

Snacks

Toasted Seeds (serves 3-4)

Packed with vitamins, minerals, protein and essential fatty acids, toasted seeds are great for snacking on. They are also good for adding to salads and soups. If possible, opt for organic and/or raw varieties.

200g/½ cup seeds such as pumpkin, sesame, sunflower and/or hemp

Generous dash of tamari or Bragg Liquid Aminos

½ teaspoon Chinese 5 Spice (optional)

¼ teaspoon chilli flakes and/or nuts such as cashew or whole almonds (optional)

Method: Add seeds, and/or nuts, to pan and dry-fry over a low heat for a few minutes. Add tamari/liquid aminos. Add spice, if using. Stir frequently until golden brown. Seeds, and nuts, toast quickly so don't leave them unattended to prevent burning. Transfer to a bowl and allow to cool.

Avocado Savoury (serves 1-2)

Rich in vitamin E, this spread is full of healthy natural oils and is good served with oatcakes, rice cakes, rye crackers or with raw vegetable cruditiés.

1 avocado
Drizzle of extra virgin olive oil
Dash of tamari or Bragg Liquid Aminos
Pinch of chilli flakes
Sea salt and freshly ground black pepper, to taste
Squeeze of fresh lemon juice (optional)

Method: Halve and peel avocado. Mash with fork. Add oil and seasonings. Serve immediately or add a squeeze of lemon juice to prevent discolouration. Eat within a few hours.

Herb Butter (approximately 15 servings)

Butter is rich in fat-soluble vitamins and, in moderation, is perfectly acceptable and preferable to commercial margarine. Serve as a spread or tossed with pasta. Alternatively, serve over baked potatoes/sweet potatoes, meat, fish or vegetables.

250g/1 cup butter (preferably organic and/or grass-fed)

Herbs such as parsley, dill, rosemary or basil

Unwaxed lemon zest, spices, chilli flakes, sea salt or freshly ground black pepper (optional)

Method: Mix butter and chopped herbs and/or additional ingredients, as desired, in a food processor and blend. Alternatively, this can be done by hand. Place on greaseproof paper, cling film or tin foil and make into a sausage shape. Place in fridge to firm. Slice and serve as required.

Tip: If dairy cannot be tolerated or if you have chosen not to eat it, this can be made using dairy-free spread.

Almond Nut Butter (approximately 20 servings)

This nutritious butter is bursting with protein and vitamin E. Full of healthy oils, it is so much better for you than processed peanut butter and tastes even better. Serve with raw vegetable cruditiés or spread on wholegrain/gluten-free bread or rice cakes. Use unsalted nuts and, if possible, organic and/or raw varieties.

300g/2 cups almonds

Drizzle of rapeseed oil (optional)

Sea salt, to taste (optional)

Method: In a food processor, grind nuts until they become a paste. If required, drizzle in a little rapeseed oil to loosen mixture. Add a pinch of salt, if using. Mix well until butter consistency is formed. Store in fridge and eat within a few days.

Tip: This also works well with other nuts such as cashews, hazelnuts and Brazil nuts. Alternatively, you can try using seeds such as sunflower and pumpkin. If you wish to reduce the presence of phytic acid, you can soak the nuts and/or seeds overnight. However, they will be very soft and this will make a moist butter that may spoil quickly. You can dehydrate them before using if you wish a more traditional texture. This produces what is known as activated nuts/seeds. You can dry them in a dehydrator for approximately 12-18 hours. Alternatively, arrange in a single layer on a baking tray and place in an oven at approximately 40-65°C/104-150°F or the lowest gas mark setting for around 12-24 hours. Dehydrate until nuts and/or seeds are dry and crisp. This is very time-consuming and is completely optional. You can also roast nuts/seeds for a richer flavour. Simply roast in an oven at 180°C/350°F/Gas Mark 4 for 10-15 minutes.

Coconut Butter (serves 3-4)

Coconut oil contains healthy fatty acids and lauric acid that helps to fight off bacterial and fungal infections. It is also good for the digestive system, immunity and skin. This coconut butter can be spread on wholegrain/gluten-free bread, crackers or oatcakes. Alternatively, serve with raw vegetable cruditiés.

100g/1 cup unsweetened desiccated coconut

1 tablespoon raw coconut oil

Pinch of sea salt

1 teaspoon raw cacao powder (optional)

Pinch of ground cinnamon (optional)

Method: Add all ingredients to a blender or food processor and blend. Keep processing until mixture becomes creamy. You may have to stop to scrape down sides of bowl to ensure even blending. Transfer ingredients to an airtight container. The coconut butter will solidify at room temperature. Simply place container in a bowl of hot water to soften.

Tip: You can also allow it to harden and cut into chunks to enjoy as a healthy snack.

Carrot, Apple and Raisins (serves 2)

Raw carrot, apple and raisins are full of beta-carotene, vitamin A, C and fibre. This makes an ideal snack and also tastes good with salads and on baked potatoes/sweet potatoes.

2 carrots, grated
1 apple, grated
Juice of ½ lemon
1 handful raisins

Method: Combine carrots and apples. Mix in raisins. Squeeze over lemon juice and mix well. Serve immediately or store in an airtight container in the fridge until ready to eat.

Bean Dip (serves 3-4)

This creamy protein-rich dip is tasty spread on rice cakes, oatcakes, wholegrain/gluten-free crackers or bread. It is also great on baked potatoes/sweet potatoes or served with raw vegetable cruditiés for dipping.

400g/14oz can cannellini beans (alternatively, use 2 cups cooked cannellini beans)

1 clove garlic, crushed or ⅛ teaspoon garlic powder

4 teaspoons extra virgin olive oil

1 teaspoon ground or 1 tablespoon fresh coriander

Sea salt and freshly ground black pepper, to taste

Method: Blend ingredients together until creamy. Store in an airtight container in fridge.

Tip: Try alternative herbs and spices such as oregano, chilli flakes or chives. Season with a herbal salt for added flavour and/or use chickpeas instead for a houmous-style dip.

Fruit, Seed and Nut Mix (serves 3-4)

This is a great snack packed full of vitamins and minerals. The dried fruit provides healthy carbohydrates and natural sugar, whilst the seeds and nuts give a protein boost and balances sugar release. Adding raw cacao nibs or carob chips adds a healthy chocolate flavour. Ideal to eat between meals, you can fill a small tub to carry with you when you are out and about. This mix is also great as a topping on porridge or yoghurt. Where possible, use organic and/or raw unsalted nuts and seeds.

1 large handful dried fruit such as chopped Medjool dates, unsulphured apricots or raisins

1 large handful seeds such as sunflower or pumpkin

1 large handful nuts such as almonds or cashews

1 large handful raw cacao nibs or unsweetened carob chips (optional)

Method: Simply combine and keep in an airtight container.

Tip: Try increasing the quantities and storing in a large, airtight container so that you always have a quick snack to hand. This recipe is not exact and you can easily replace the fruit, seeds and nuts for others of your choice.

About The Authors

Sharon Pitman and Lorraine Pitman are sisters and co-founders of Holistichem. Both have a passion for wellbeing and enjoy writing and sharing their knowledge on integrating positive changes to diet and lifestyle.

They are both complementary therapists qualified in stress management and relaxation therapies. Sharon is also qualified in all advanced aspects of Holistic Nutrition. Lorraine has an interest in nutrition too, having successfully undertaken study in Food Intolerances and Allergies and alongside Sharon, uses this knowledge to develop their low-allergen, clean eating recipes.

Together, they developed the Holistichem Wellbeing Method. For Sharon, this provided a holistic way of coping with, and improving, her personal experience of chronic illness. For Lorraine, this has helped to improve her health and wellbeing.

They have a keen interest in the link between creativity and wellbeing and also create a range of handmade wellbeing jewellery.

To find out more, visit www.holistichem.com.

Sharon and Lorraine were both born and bred in Scotland. They live in Erskine, just outside Glasgow.